THE TMJ BOOK

THE TMJ BOOK

Andrew S. Kaplan, D.M.D.,
and Gray Williams, Jr.

•

Illustrations by Caroline Meinstein
Medical Arts Department, The Mount Sinai Hospital

PHAROS BOOKS
A SCRIPPS HOWARD COMPANY
NEW YORK

First published in 1988.

Library of Congress Cataloging-in-Publication Data:
Kaplan, Andrew, 1956-
The TMJ book.

Includes index.
1. Temporomandibular joint—Diseases. I. Williams, Gray, 1932- . II. Title.
RK470.K37 1988 617'.522 88-42720
ISBN 0-88687-358-4

Printed in the United States of America.

Pharos Books
A Scripps Howard Company
200 Park Avenue
New York, Ny 10166

10 9 8 7 6 5 4 3 2

Cover and interior design: Elyse Strongin

To our wives, Sandra and Marian,
and our children.

CONTENTS

THE TMJ BOOK

ACKNOWLEDGMENTS

In this book, we emphasize that treating temporomandibular joint disorders often requires the collaboration of experts from several different fields. The same is true of writing this book. Gray Williams and I owe an enormous debt of gratitude to many of my professional colleagues, who have given generously of their time and knowledge to help us assure the accuracy and comprehensiveness of our work.

First of all, we owe thanks to attending staff members of the TMJ clinic at Mt. Sinai, who provided much of the specialized information in this text. Dr. Jay Goldman supplied us with invaluable information on trauma-related disorders and on the complexities of insurance, based upon his extensive experience in treating accident victims. Much of the chapter on treatment of psychological stress resulted from consultations with the psychologist on our team, Dr. Andrew Elmore. Dr. Gordon Gaynor provided us with the basis of the section on the use of orthodontics in phase-two TMJ treatment. And Dr. Arthur Elias, chief of oral surgery at Mt. Sinai, supplied us with much of the information on open-joint and orthognathic surgery. All of these individuals not only assisted in the original research for our work, but were good enough to review it carefully and to make many excellent suggestions for its improvement.

Likewise, two other colleagues were of great help both in providing original information and in later, painstaking review. Oral and maxillofacial surgeon Dr. Howard Israel of the Columbia University School of Dentistry generously supplied us with details of his experience and research in the field of arthroscopic surgery. John Dunn,

L.P.T., similarly provided us with up-to-date information on the use of physical therapy in TMJ treatment.

We would also like to thank several other colleagues who read the manuscript and offered very useful comments and suggestions. These include Dr. Michael Gelb, director of research at the TMJ and facial pain clinic at the University of Medicine and Dentistry of New Jersey; Dr. Steven Syrop, director of the TMJ and facial pain clinic at Columbia University School of Dentistry; Dr. Kenneth Aschheim and Dr. J. Gordon Rubin, members of the attending staff in the dental department at Mt. Sinai; Dr. Jack Klatell, chairman and director of the dental department; and Lourdes Guerrero, my dental assistant. And we owe a debt of gratitude to Dr. Daniel Buchbinder of Mt. Sinai for his advice on the illustrations.

I would like to express my personal appreciation to those who encouraged me to develop my interest in this field. First, I want to thank my father, a "wet-finger" dentist (as we say in the profession), whose own early interest in TMJ disorders originally stimulated mine. I would also like to express my gratitude to Dr. Noshir Mehta, director of the Gelb Facial-Pain Clinic at Tufts University School of Dental Medicine, and to Dr. Albert Forgione, also of Tufts, who encouraged my curiosity as a young research assistant, trying to learn about what was then a fairly new and mysterious subject. Dr. Harold Gelb, one of the pioneers in TMJ treatment, taught me much and provided me with valued encouragement and support. And a special thank you goes to Dr. Klatell, who provided me with the opportunity to direct the TMJ clinic at Mt. Sinai, and who has always kept the door open for advice and guidance.

Thanks must also be given to my patients, several of whom graciously consented to be interviewed for this book. It is from working with them that I have learned the most about this complex and challenging field. And of course, there is nothing more satisfying than to use one's knowledge and experience in relieving patients' pain and remedying their disorders.

Appreciation is also due to the many researchers and clinicians who, over the past several decades, have established the foundations for the diagnosis and treatment of TMJ disorders, and have been particularly influential in disseminating this information through their teaching and writing. It is unfortunately impossible to acknowledge all these leaders here, but a few deserve special mention: the late Dr. Nathan Allen Shore of New York City, who was an early explorer of the relationship between occlusion and TMJ disorders, as well as other aspects of the TMJ; the late Dr. Laszlo Schwartz of Columbia University School of Dentistry, who directed one of the first TMJ clinics and who is especially known for research connecting TMJ disorders with psychological stress; Dr. Parker Mahan of the University of Florida at Gainesville, who, over a long period, has been a leading researcher into many aspects of the TMJ anatomy and its disorders; Dr. William Sollberg, director of the TMJ clinic at UCLA, another wide-ranging researcher whose studies have been important in clarifying the structure and mechanics of the joint and the disorders that afflict it; the late Dr. William Farrar and his colleague Dr. William McCarty, both of Montgomery, Alabama, whose pioneering clinical investigations have led to the understanding of disk dislocation; Dr. Janet Travell, famed for her work on musuclar pain and the dynamics of muscle trigger points; radiologist Richard Katzberg, M.D., of the University of Rochester Medical Center, who has made important contributions in the use of X-rays and other imaging techniques to diagnose TMJ disorders; John Rugh, Ph.D., of the University of Texas at San Antonio, noted for his research on the relationship between muscle activity and other facets of

TMJ function; Dr. Peter Dawson of St. Petersburg, Florida, a prosthodontist who has demonstrated the usefulness of restorative dentistry in giving long-range relief for TMJ disorders; Dr. Brendan Stack of Springfield, Virginia, who has done much to disseminate information on the use of orthodontics to treat TMJ disorders; Dr. Franklin Dolwick of the University of Florida, whose research, teaching, and writing have significantly contributed to progress in the use of oral surgery to treat TMJ problems; Dr. Bruce Sanders of UCLA, co-author with Dr. Dolwick of an important and influential text on TMJ surgery and also noted for his clinical work in arthroscopic surgery; Dr. Joseph McCain of Miami, Florida, another pioneer in the clinical use of arthroscopic surgery for the treatment of TMJ disorders; Dr. Welden Bell of the University of Texas Southwest Medical School, Dr. Jeffrey Okeson of the University of Kentucky, Dr. Harold Gelb of the University of Medicine and Dentistry of New Jersey, and Dr. Mark Friedman of Mt. Vernon, New York, each of whom has used his research and clinical experience to develop a current professional text on TMJ disorders.

Finally, Gray and I would like to express our gratitude to the publishing professionals who have made this book a reality: Editor-in-Chief Hana Lane and Assistant Editor Sharilyn Jee of Pharos Books, for their careful evaluation and supervision of every stage of production; copy editor Herb Kirk, for his meticulous attention to detail and impeccable editorial taste; and our literary agent, Michael Cohn, for his encouragement and judicious counsel, from gleam-in-the-eye to published book.

Andrew S. Kaplan

ONE

THE PAINFUL PRETENDERS

Like many patients on their first visit, Joy Forrester was in evident pain. "I've had headaches all my life," she told me, "but nothing like this." During the past month she had become more and more incapacitated. Sometimes the pain seemed to radiate outward from behind her eyes and into her cheeks. Sometimes it shot upward from her temples to the top of her head. Lately pain and ringing had developed in her ears as well.

At first she thought her allergies were acting up and inflaming her sinuses. As she put it, "I am allergic to everything I breathe." She received year-round shots and a variety of drugs to keep her symptoms under control. So she went first to her allergist, who prescribed a powerful steroid medication to reduce inflammation. It didn't work. Rather, as steroids often do, it irritated her digestive tract and had to be quickly abandoned. Then began a procession of visits to several other baffled physicians, while the pain grew steadily worse.

She saw a neurologist, a gynecologist, an internist, an ear-nose-throat specialist (otolaryngolist), and another allergist. Severe chronic headaches are among the most difficult of all symptoms to treat successfully, since they can have so many different causes. All these physicians could do for her was eliminate one possible diagnosis after another. Nor was her morale helped by lightly veiled suggestions that her pain might be merely psychological.

Finally, after performing the usual tests and hearing her history, the second allergist concluded that her problem wasn't an allergy. "In fact," he told her, "just about all the usual reasons for your headaches appear to have been considered. But there is one other possibility."

"What's that?"

"You may be suffering from a TMJ disorder." She had never heard of it.

"Let me show you what I mean."

The allergist placed his fingertips on the sides of her face, just in front of her ears, and pressed lightly. "I almost passed out from the pain," she reported. The doctor explained that the tender areas were in the joints that connected her lower jaw to her skull: the temporomandibular joints, or TMJs. "TMJ disorders aren't usually treated by physicians," he said. "They're treated by dentists."

And that's how she eventually came to my office. I am one of a growing number of dentists who concentrate largely on the treatment of TMJ disorders. They make up the bulk of my work, both in private practice and at the Mount Sinai Medical Center TMJ clinic in New York, of which I am director. My colleagues and I see several hundred TMJ patients each year.

Many of them have never heard of the TMJ, much less TMJ disorders. And they don't associate their problems with their jaws. Joy Forrester's first symptoms, remember, were blinding headaches. Often these patients go looking vainly for help from one physician to another, and the physicians either don't know what the problem is or can't treat it successfully.

Their main complaint is pain—pain that is often persistent, agonizing, and debilitating. The pain may occasionally subside, giving the sufferer the illusion that it is gone for good, only to reappear, often worse than ever, days, weeks, or months later. It may vary during the day: for some it is worse in the morning, for others in the afternoon or evening. For some it is relentless and unremitting, all day and every day. Painkillers and other drugs give little or no relief, and the side effects sometimes make matters worse.

The emotional suffering is perhaps even worse than the physical. As they continue to suffer, these patients become absorbed in their pain: it takes over their lives. Many become unable to work or to cope with the ordinary tasks of living. One patient admitted to me in mortification that she had virtually handed over her small children to the care of a neighbor. She just couldn't manage her household and her pain at the same time.

The sufferers feel isolated and alone. Their self-absorbed misery inevitably frays the sympathy and patience even of those most dear to them. The symptoms are not visible—you can't *see* someone else's pain. As a result, marriages become strained or broken, families become alienated, friendships drop away.

The suffering is often reinforced by frustrating medical experiences. Many physicians either give up or prescribe treatment that is ineffective. Frequently they are urged to seek psychiatric help in the mistaken belief that their problems are "all in their heads."

Not surprisingly, these people also suffer from low self-confidence and self-esteem. They come to experience their debilitating pain as a sign of personal weakness and failure. As one patient put it, "It's hard to feel good about yourself when your body is giving you so much grief."

TMJ-disorder pain is deceptive. It baffles many health professionals, and it certainly baffles the unfortunate patients. It doesn't have to be located in or near the joint at all. Joy Forrester's headaches are typical, but there are many other examples.

For instance, a middle-aged woman made five visits to the Mount Sinai dental clinic complaining of a persistent ache in one of her molars. But there was nothing wrong with the tooth that anyone could find—no decay, no abscess, no painful sensitivity to tapping or to heat or cold. The dental residents were prepared to start root-canal treatment, hoping it would relieve her pain, but one of them asked me to take a look first.

I found a small, hard knot of muscle in the middle of the woman's cheek. I asked the resident for the lidocaine syringe with which he was about to anesthetize the tooth. I injected a small amount of anesthetic into the knot of muscle. In less than a minute, a look of astonishment came over the woman's face. "The pain is gone," she said. "This is the first time in two months that tooth hasn't hurt!"

The tooth wasn't the source of her pain at all. The pain was *referred* to the tooth, from the area of constricted muscle. And the muscle constriction was in turn caused by a TMJ disorder. Eventually we were able to relieve all her problems.

Another typical example: A young woman was referred to the clinic by an ear-nose-throat specialist. She had gone to him with a severe earache, but he could find no sign of infection or any other problem with her ear. Fortunately he was familiar with TMJ disorders and their capacity for producing symptoms elsewhere. So he sent her to us. We were not surprised to find that she had a nervous habit of grinding her teeth and that her jaw made a noticeable clicking sound when she opened and closed it. Further examination confirmed a TMJ disorder. Treating it soon got rid of her earache.

One more common problem. A young man suffered whiplash injuries to his neck and back in an auto accident. He received physical therapy for strain to these muscles, and after six weeks felt almost fully recovered. Then he suddenly began to suffer severe headaches behind one eye and down the side of his face.

At first he didn't associate these problems with the accident. The lawyer handling his insurance claim knew that accidents often cause TMJ disorders and referred him to us. We were able to establish that the whiplash had caused damage to one of the TMJs, indirectly causing pain in the head and facial muscles. Again, getting rid of the pain required treating the TMJ disorder.

These patients are typical. In each case, the TMJ disorder played the role of a "painful pretender," displaying symptoms that could easily be blamed on some other ailment. Such symptoms include:

- *Headaches,* often severe and recurrent. They tend to occur more commonly on one side than on both and in areas around the eyes, cheeks, and temples, but they can also occur at the top or base of the skull.
- *Toothaches* that cannot be traced to decay, nerve death, or inflammation.
- *Burning, tingling sensations,* especially in the tongue but sometimes in the mouth or throat.
- *Earaches* or "stuffed" sensations in the ears, sometimes accompanied by dizziness, or by ringing or rushing noises.
- *Neckaches or shoulderaches,* sometimes accompanied by numbness in the arms or hands.
- *Tenderness and swelling,* particularly in the sides of the face.

• *Clicking or popping noises* when opening the jaw, closing it, or both.

• *Inability to open the mouth freely*, either because of pain, or because some impediment seems to "lock" the jaw at a certain point. If the problem occurs on one side only, the jaw may not open straight but slides off to one side.

TMJ disorders tend to afflict more women than men, by a ratio of about four to one. Nobody knows why, and a good deal of research is currently being devoted to the question. (Other ailments behave this way, too. Gout, for example, afflicts more men than women, rheumatoid arthritis more women than men.)

Reviewing the cases of the thousands of TMJ patients that my colleagues and I have observed over the years gave me the idea for this book. TMJ disorders are extremely common. Statistical studies suggest that about 5 percent of the population suffers from them to one degree or another. That's one person in twenty, or about 10 million Americans. Some people are not severely troubled, and some learn to live with the discomfort. But many are afflicted seriously enough to be incapacitated, particularly by the pain that is the most common symptom. Much of this suffering is unnecessary.

At the same time, TMJ disorders remain among the most misunderstood of human ailments. Although they are essentially medical problems (and certainly have medical symptoms), they are usually treated by dentists, and a minority of dentists at that. Only rather recently have many physicians, dentists, and other health professionals become well enough informed even to diagnose them correctly. A few still don't know how to recognize these conditions or what treatment to recommend.

One reason for this confusion is the fact that TMJ disorders are not only confusing but also complex. They have several basic causes and exhibit a wide range of symptoms. Moreover, even though dentists may provide the basic treatment, the cooperation of others—physicians, oral surgeons, therapists of several kinds—is necessary for satisfactory long-range results.

This book is designed to take the mystery out of TMJ disorders, especially for those who suffer from them or have reason to think they might. I will explain, with as little technical language as possible, just what the problems are, how to determine whether you might be suffering from one of them, and what can be done to treat them. The following chapters will answer questions like these:

- What is the TMJ, and how does it work?
- What goes wrong with it—and why?
- Where can I go for help?
- What kinds of treatment are available? What are they intended to achieve? What are their chances of success?
- How much does treatment cost? Will health insurance cover it?
- What can I do to help myself? How can I relieve TMJ symptoms?
- How can I reduce my chances of getting a TMJ disorder in the first place?

Throughout I have drawn on my own experiences as well as those of my colleagues at Mount. Sinai. The case histories in this book are real, although the names of our patients and some details have been changed to protect their privacy. There is nothing unique about the approaches and procedures described here. The same methods, or ones very like them, are used widely and successfully by other TMJ practitioners and their associates over much of the world.

Above all, this book offers hope. Not every TMJ disorder can be treated successfully. Not every success is 100 percent complete. But a large percentage of cases *can* be helped. Pain can be eliminated or significantly reduced and quality of life markedly improved. If this book helps you to understand these problems better, and to find treatment that works for you, you will have satisfied my main purpose in writing it.

TWO

The TMJ

HOW IT WORKS

"You definitely have tenderness in the left masseter and medial pterygoid," I told the patient. "You also have a history of clenching, and persistent clicking. All these suggest an articular disk derangement."

The patient looked completely baffled. "Left master *what?*"

"I'm sorry," I said. "Let me explain . . . ."

I should have known better. Before anyone can understand what causes TMJ disorders, some basic anatomy must be made clear, so I'll explain it here. I won't go into much detail, but you need to know some of the parts of the body involved and to be reasonably familiar with their names.

These names may at first seem rather forbidding—they are basically Greek and Latin words scientists have used for centuries to make sure they're all talking about the same things. But once you know what the words mean in plain English, they're not hard to understand. They are the terms that I will be using throughout this book and that your own dentist or physician is likely to use in discussing your condition with you.

• The Bones of the TMJ

We'll start with the bones that meet at the joint. (Refer to Figures 1 through 3.)

The human skull has two main components: the *cranium* and the *mandible*. The cranium is an assembly of several bones bound (or *sutured*) together to form a single unit. Two of these components are the *temporal bones*—the bones of the temples, one on each side of the head.

Mandible comes from a Latin word meaning "to chew." The mandible is in fact the U-shaped jawbone you use to chew with. At each end it forms a flexible joint with one of the temporal bones of the cranium. In simple English this might be called a jaw joint, but the precise medical term is *temporomandibular joint*, which is mercifully shortened to *TMJ*.

On each end of the mandible, at the joint, is an enlarged,

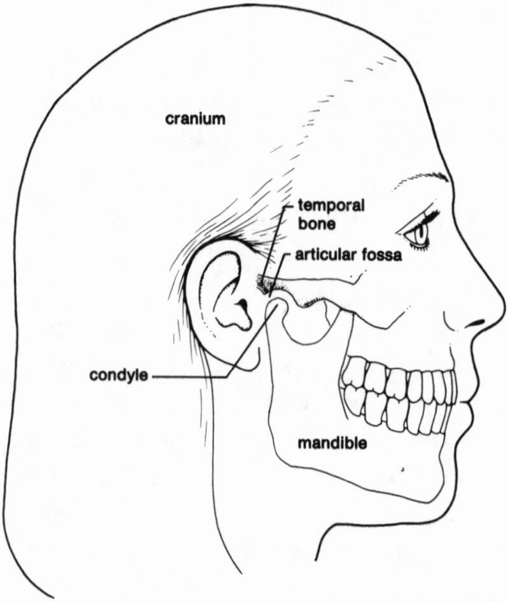

Figure 1. The bones of the temporomandibular joint (TMJ). When the mouth is closed, the condyle on each end of the mandible is located in the hollow of the articular fossa.

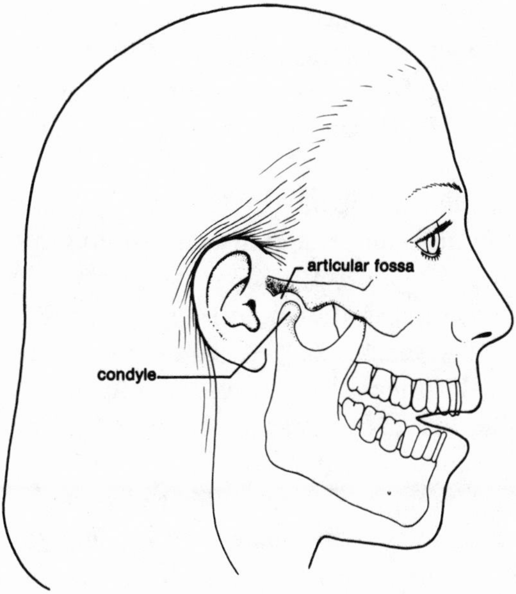

Figure 2. As the mouth begins to open, the condyle rotates within the fossa.

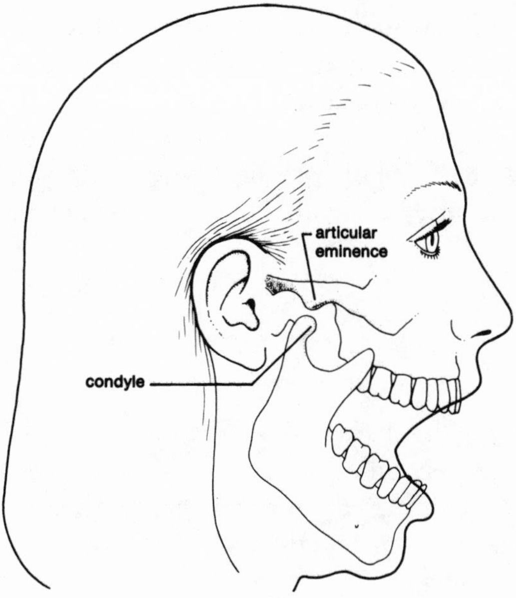

Figure 3. But as the mouth opens fully, the condyle translates—slides down and forward—toward the lowest point of the articular eminence. When the mouth closes, the process is reversed.

smooth, rounded protrusion called a *condyle* (pronounced KON-dile; from a Greek word meaning "knob"). When the jaw is closed, the condyle fits into a rounded hollow of the temporal bone called the *articular fossa* (from Latin words meaning "joint" and "ditch").

You might suppose that as the mouth opens and the jaw drops, the rounded condyle at each end would simply rotate within the rounded fossa. But that wouldn't provide enough range of motion for the mouth to open fully. When opening begins, each condyle does rotate (as shown in Figure 2). But then it also *translates*—it moves from one place to another. As you can see in Figure 3, the condyle moves down and forward out of the fossa, toward a rounded bump on the temporal bone called the *articular eminence*. You can actually feel this movement if you press your fingers lightly on the areas directly in front of your ears and then open your mouth wide.

That's a lot of movement for a joint to make, and indeed the TMJ is one of the loosest and most flexible joints in the whole body. This flexibility enables you to take big bites of your food and then chew it thoroughly. It also helps you stand erect, with your head up, and to eat and swallow without your neck and jaw getting in the way of each other. Finally, the flexibility of the TMJ helps make it possible for you to utter the wide range of sounds you need for speech.

• The Soft Tissues

The movements of the TMJ are both facilitated and limited by what are collectively called *soft tissues*. Most of them aren't really soft at all—they're just not as hard as bone.

One of the most important functions of soft tissue is to *lubricate* the joint, reducing the friction that would occur if the hard bones rubbed directly against one another. For instance, in all the joints of the body, including the TMJ, the bearing areas of the bones are coated with pliable *cartilage*. This acts as a kind of shock absorber and provides a smoother, slicker surface than bone.

But the TMJ has in addition a separate, specialized piece of fibrous cartilage that sits like a slippery cushion between the condyle and the temporal bone (see Figure 4). It is called the *articular disk*. It isn't completely round, but shaped like a broad crescent, so it is also called a *meniscus*, from a Greek word for the crescent moon. The ends of the crescent point downward along the sides of the condyle. Between these ends, the disk is divided longitudinally into three segments. The middle segment is considerably thinner than those in front and behind. The cartilage

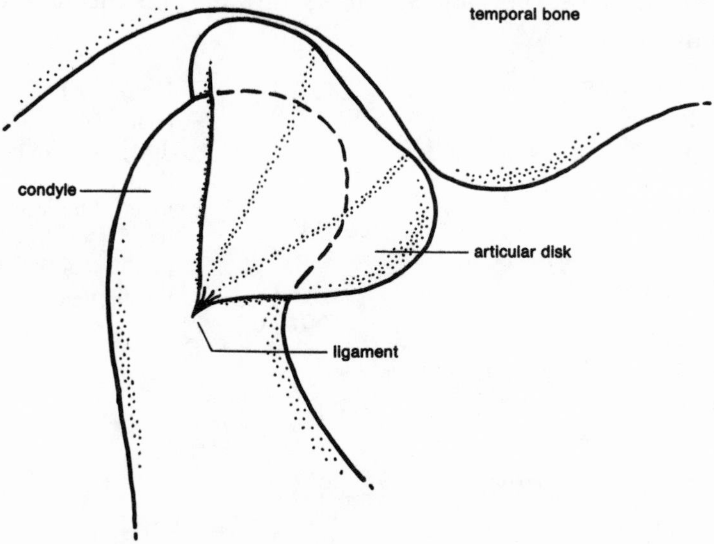

Figure 4. The crescent-shaped articular disk forms a cushion of flexible cartilage between the condyle and the temporal bone. It is attached to the condyle with short ligaments, and is composed of three segments—the middle one thinner than the other two.

of the disk is flexible enough to bend and flatten in the varying space between the bones, as the condyle translates out of the fossa and along the eminence.

The bones of the joint, and the articular disk, must not only move freely and smoothly but also must be kept from drifting too far apart. This second function is performed mainly by the tough connective tissues called *ligaments.* Ligaments on the points of the articular disk, for instance, attach it to the condyle so it won't slip off to either side. Other ligaments extending between the cranium and mandible (Figure 5) limit and control the movement of the jaw so it won't open too wide or become otherwise dislocated.

And some ligaments form a cylindrical web, the *capsule,* that surrounds the whole joint. The capsule contains a lining called the *synovium* which produces slippery *synovial fluid.* This fluid fills the empty spaces inside the capsule and coats the bearing surfaces, further lubricating the joint.

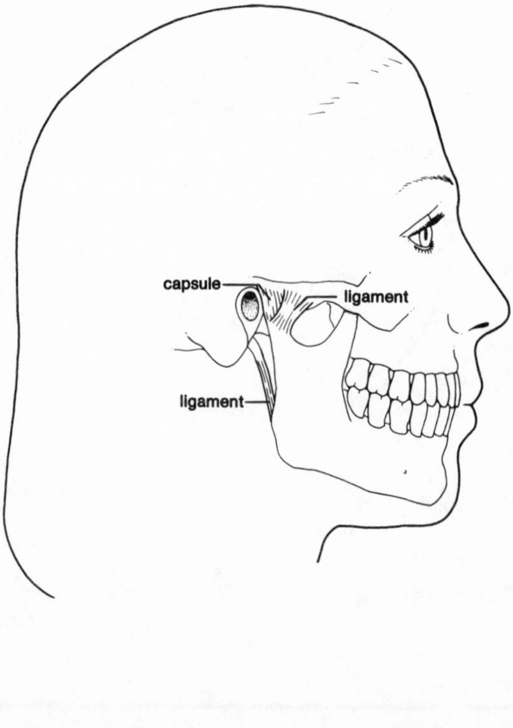

Figure 5. The ligaments of the TMJ limit and control its movement. The joint itself is enclosed in a capsule of ligament-like tissue.

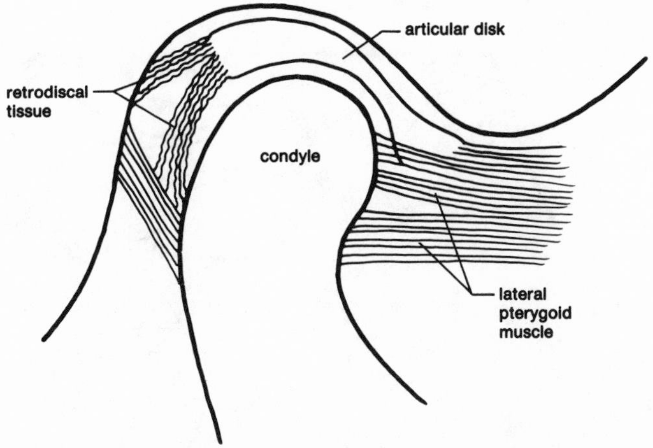

Figure 6. Inside the capsule, the articular disk (seen here in cross-section) is connected to the temporal bone behind it by retrodiscal tissue. When the mouth is closed, the retrodiscal tissue is folded and compressed.

Inside the capsule (Figure 6), just behind the disk, is connective tissue called (from its location) *retrodiscal tissue*. Part of it is composed of ligaments connecting the disk to the temporal bone and the condyle. But much of it is a fairly loose, spongy material. Unlike most other parts of the joint, it contains many blood vessels and nerves. This is the tissue that bleeds most easily and is most sensitive to pain. Both of these facts are important, as you will see in the chapters to come.

Also crucial are the working relationships between the hard tissues—the bones—and the soft tissues, particularly the disk and the retrodiscal tissue. As shown in Figure 7, the soft tissues shift and bend as the lower jaw opens and closes. The retrodiscal tissue is folded and compressed in the joint space when the jaw is closed. Then, when the jaw opens and the condyle moves down and forward, the retrodiscal tissue stretches out and helps stabilize the disk on the condyle.

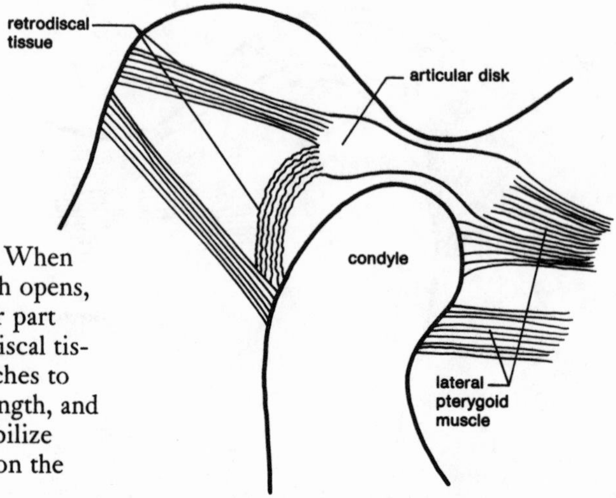

Figure 7. When the mouth opens, the upper part of retrodiscal tissue stretches to its full length, and helps stabilize the disk on the condyle.

• The Chewing Muscles

The movements of the TMJ are produced by the chewing muscles—known formally as the *muscles of mastication*—running between the cranium and mandible on each side of the head. They are said to *originate* on the fixed cranium and to *insert* on the moving mandible. They are attached to the bones by connective tissue known as *tendons*.

A muscle can exert force in only one direction. It can only pull, or *contract*. It cannot push; it can only *relax*. Different sets of muscles are thus required for the opposite movements of the mandible: one set for opening, another set for closure; one set to move the jaw forward, another to move it back. The muscles that produce forward movement are also used, alternately, to move the jaw from side to side. Because so many TMJ problems involve the muscles, it is helpful to know some of their names and how they work.

To provide the force needed for chewing, the muscles

for closing the jaw are stronger than those needed to open it. There are three closing muscles on each side. Figure 8 shows one of these—the *masseter* ("chewer" in Greek). It originates on the temporal bone and extends down the outside of the mandible to its lower back corner, or angle. You can easily feel it contracting and relaxing under the skin if you lightly press your fingers against your lower cheek near the angle while opening and closing your mouth.

The second muscle (see Figure 9) parallels the masseter on the inside of the jaw. It is called the *medial pterygoid* muscle because it originates at a wing-shaped protrusion of the cranium (*pterygoid* comes from a Greek term meaning "shaped like a wing"). The masseter and medial pterygoid muscles form a sort of sling around the angle of the mandible and work together to pull it shut.

The third closing muscle (Figure 10) looks like a partly spread fan on the side of the head. Its broad end originates

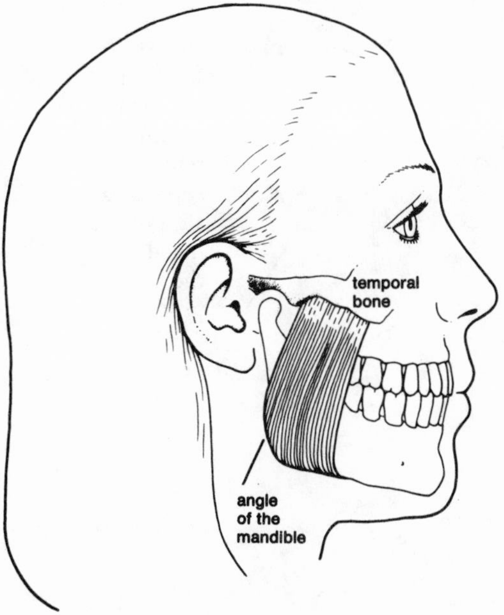

Figure 8. The strongest of the muscles of mastication is the masseter, or "chewer," which originates on the temporal bone, and inserts on the angle of the mandible.

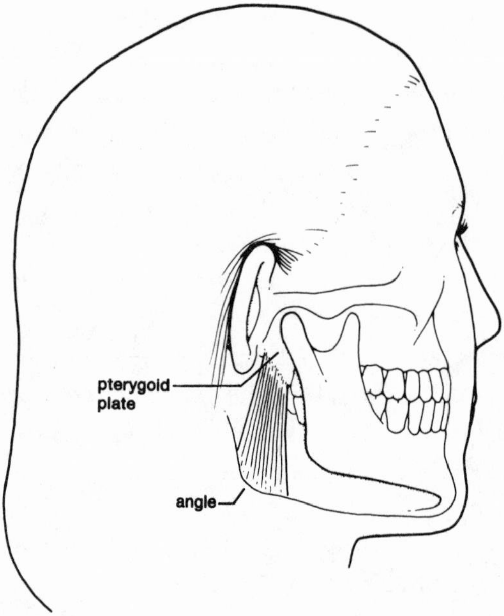

Figure 9. One of the medial pterygoid muscles, viewed from inside the jaws. It originates on a protrusion of the cranium called the pterygoid plate, and inserts on the inside of the angle, forming a kind of sling with the masseter.

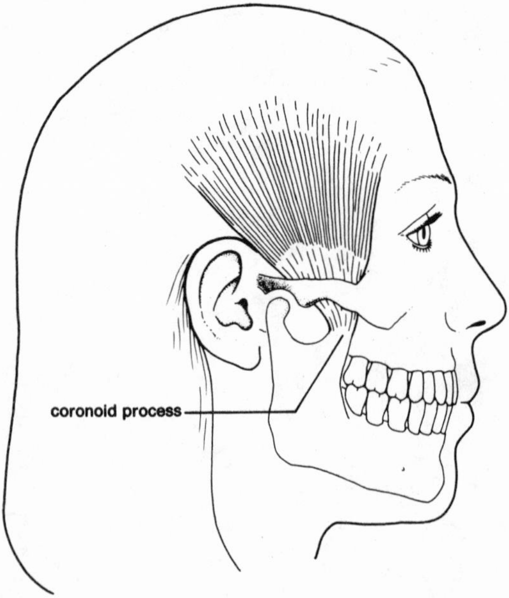

Figure 10. The fan-shaped temporalis muscle originates on the temple, and inserts on a protrusion of the mandible called the coronoid process.

high on the temple, so it is called the *temporalis* muscle. Its narrow end inserts on the mandible in front of the condyle, on a secondary protrusion called the *coronoid process*. The temporalis, like the masseter, is a muscle that you can feel working. As you open and shut your mouth, press your fingers lightly against your temples in front of and just above your ears. You will feel the temporalis muscles on each side shifting under the skin.

The muscles for opening the jaw, known as *accessory* muscles of mastication, are mainly located under the chin. They are less likely to be involved in TMJ disorders than the closing muscles, so it isn't important for you to know their individual names and functions.

When you chew, you move your jaw not only up and down but also forward and back and side to side. These movements are largely produced by the pair of *lateral pterygoid* muscles (Figure 11). They originate at the same re-

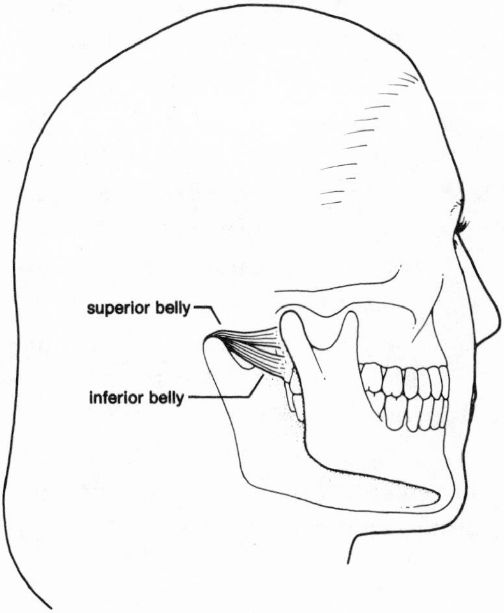

Figure 11. The superior and inferior bellies of the lateral pterygoid muscles, viewed from inside the jaws. They originate on the pterygoid plate, and extend back and outward to the condyle. The superior belly is connected both to the condyle and to the disk, and partly controls the position of the disk (see also *Figures 6* and *7*).

gions of the cranium as the medial pterygoid muscles and extend backward and outward (laterally) toward the condyles. Each was once thought to be a single muscle, but we now know that the upper (*superior*) part works differently from the lower (*inferior*) part. So the parts are given two separate names: they are called the *superior belly* and the *inferior belly* of the lateral pterygoid muscle (see Figures 6 and 7).

The pair of inferior bellies is the one mainly responsible for moving the jaw forward. When these bellies contract they pull the condyles forward out of the fossae and down to the lowest points of the eminences. (You can produce this movement voluntarily by opening your mouth slightly and jutting your jaw forward. The movement also takes place spontaneously when the mouth is opened wide.) The inferior bellies, contracting alternately one at a time, are also responsible for moving the jaw from side to side.

The superior bellies work differently. For one thing, each one is not simply attached to the mandible. Instead, some of its fibers pass through the the joint capsule and connect with the front of the articular disk inside. The superior belly contracts only when the jaw is *closing*—just the opposite of the inferior belly. It then exerts forward pressure on both condyle and disk, apparently stabilizing their relationship to each other and assuring that they will be in the most effective position possible when the strong force of chewing moves the condyle backward and upward. Dysfunction of this muscle is related to one very common kind of TMJ disorder.

Other muscles, particularly in the neck and back, connect directly or indirectly with the chewing muscles and interact with them. I describe them in more detail in Chapter 6.

• The Nerves of the TMJ

Both control and sensation in the TMJ are provided by nerves—the nerves of the joint itself and of the neighboring regions of the head—that are arranged like the trunk and branches of a tree. The trunk is the *trigeminal* nerve, which has three main branches (*trigeminal* comes from a word meaning "triplets"). One of these branches, the *mandibular*, spreads into the area of the mandible. One of the mandibular branch that penetrates the TMJ itself is called the *auriculotemporal nerve—atn* for short.

Knowing the names of the nerves is perhaps less important than knowing what nerves, in general, do. Nerves are made up of parallel strands of long thin cells called *neurons*. There are two kinds of neurons and they have separate functions. One is that of the *motor* nerves: the nerves that control how tissues such as muscles act. The other kind is that of *sensory* nerves: the nerves that feel. Sensory neurons have a variety of specialized endings to feel particular things—position, say, or pressure, or pain.

Of course, pain especially concerns us here. The specialized neuron endings for pain respond only when they are stimulated in certain ways. The stimulus might be damage to the nerve itself or to the tissue around it. Or it might be a chemical change in the surrounding tissue, of the kind that results from fatigue or inflammation. In any event, the stimulated neuron relays the pain "message" through a chain of other neurons to the central nervous system—the spinal cord and the brain.

In the brain, the pain sensation is processed in various ways. For example, the pain is made *conscious:* you become aware of how severe it is and where it is located. But here something can happen that is very puzzling and not well understood. The brain may interpret the sensation as coming from somewhere else. The pain is said to be *referred* from its true source to some other part of the body.

That is why I call TMJ disorders "the painful pretenders." Disorders in and around the temporomandibular joint very often produce referred pain somewhere else—a headache, an earache, a toothache, or a pain in the neck.

• The Teeth

The chief function of all the structures I've described is *chewing:* moving the teeth into proper positions for cutting food up and grinding it down so it can be swallowed and digested. The teeth themselves, and their placement in relation to one another (Figure 12), have a powerful effect on the other parts of the mechanism.

Ideally, the teeth are aligned so that when the jaws are closed, the cutting teeth—the *incisors* and *canines*—in the upper jaw slightly overlap those in the lower. All the milling teeth—the *premolars* and *molars*—in one jaw should then make even contact with those in the other jaw. The

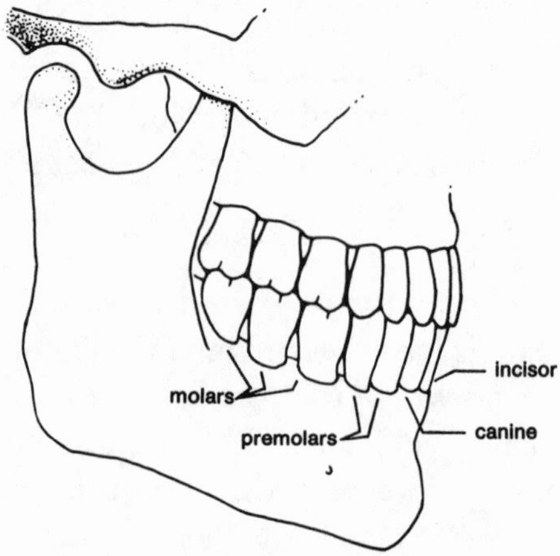

Figure 12. The teeth. The incisors in front are flanked on each side by canine teeth. Behind these, on each side of each jaw, are two premolars. And behind those are three molars. The last of the molars are sometimes called wisdom teeth.

highest points (or *cusps*) of the lower teeth should mesh with the hollows in the upper ones.

That's the ideal. But there is enormous genetic variability in human teeth. They can be too big, or too small, for the jaws they rest in, and they often grow in crookedly. Moreover, the jaws themselves may be mismatched: one may be much larger or smaller than the other. And then things happen to teeth. They get cavities. They get broken. Some or all may eventually have to be removed. As a result, a bad bite, or *malocclusion*, is more common than not.

Malocclusion reduces chewing efficiency. If that were its only consequence, it would be tolerable in most cases. Unfortunately, it can throw the whole chewing mechanism out of balance. And that, as you will see, is an important source of TMJ disorders.

THREE

The TMJ

WHAT CAN GO WRONG

We've just seen how the TMJ works—or, rather, how it ought to work. Unfortunately, a number of things can go wrong, mainly because of its complexity and the precise interdependence of its parts.

First of all, the joint is very loose, with a wide range of movement, and it requires specialized tissues like the articular disk to keep it moving smoothly. The mandible, in fact, doesn't rest on anything solid; it is suspended by the delicately balanced forces of its muscles.

The teeth are another potential source of trouble. They should meet evenly when they bite, but they are fragile and often irregular.

Finally, if any single component fails to function properly, the others have trouble compensating. Indeed, a seemingly minor malfunction in one part can lead to serious problems in the others.

Moreover, TMJ problems are almost never single problems. They often have multiple, overlapping causes—causes that are hard to pin down exactly. And they often have multiple, overlapping effects as well. So there is no single, "magic" treatment that works in every case. My colleagues and I at Mount Sinai have found that a wide range of approaches is needed, and close cooperation with experts in several different fields. I call TMJ disorders multifactorial problems, which require multidisciplinary solutions.

So, if you ask "What *exactly* causes TMJ disorders?" I have to reply "I don't know." I would be extremely skeptical of anyone who claims that he or she *does* know. The subject is one of much research, and the experts don't always agree. Nevertheless, two often interrelated factors appear to be the causes of many TMJ problems. These are malocclusion of the teeth and psychological stress. In addition, a third factor often seems to be a contributing cause—bad postural habits, particularly of the head and neck. And finally, there are two special, "outside" causes. One is trauma: direct physical injury, as from an accident. The other is disease, such as rheumatoid arthritis, which can produce TMJ pain among its other symptoms.

• Malocclusion

Very few people have "perfect" teeth; the ideal model I described earlier is usually just that. Moreover, malocclusion—even severe malocclusion—doesn't inevitably result in a TMJ disorder. The human body has a remarkable ability to adjust to imperfections and abnormalities of all sorts, and most people with malocclusion suffer nothing more serious than diminished efficiency in chewing.

Nonetheless, malocclusion not only appears to be an important cause of TMJ disorders in itself, it also contributes to those that have other causes. Sometimes the defective bite is congenital or of long standing, producing TMJ problems only after many years. Sometimes it occurs rather suddenly—losing teeth, especially on just one side, is a common precipitating circumstance.

I hate to admit it, but dental treatment, especially restorative treatment, can also be responsible. Caps or crowns that are too high or low throw the bite off balance. So, sometimes, does orthodontic treatment, especially if the teeth are straightened cosmetically without taking the relationship of the TMJs into account. Fortunately, more and more dentists are becoming familiar with TMJ problems and can prevent such problems from occurring.

But whatever its origin, malocclusion puts a strain on the TMJ—the joint itself and its muscles. The main chewing muscles—masseters, pterygoids, and temporalis muscles (see Figures 8 through 11)—tend to suffer the most. During chewing, the teeth automatically seek a position that provides the most powerful bite under the circumstances. If the bite is uneven—from front to back, or side to side—the muscles cannot work harmoniously. Instead, some must work harder than others. In the process they can become overworked and fatigued.

If you've ever suffered muscle cramp, such as a charley horse or a shinsplint, you know that a fatigued muscle can become stiff and sore. When the muscle is overworked, lactic acid builds up in it and it tends to go into prolonged contraction, sometimes called muscle spasm. At the same time, the nerves in the muscle register pain.

So, overworked, fatigued chewing muscles may become aching or tender, and small, perpetually taut areas eventually form within them. These *trigger points* can occur in any muscle. (The term was coined by Dr. Janet Travell, who is probably best known for treating President John F. Kennedy's bad back.) Trigger points may or may not be painful themselves, but they serve to set off referred muscle pain elsewhere in the body. In fact, trigger points appear essential to the whole phenomenon of referred pain described in Chapter 2.

Moreover, the fatigued chewing muscles create other problems. If you've ever sprained your ankle, you know that your other muscles automatically tend to favor it. You limp, to avoid putting painful pressure on the injured part. This *muscle guarding* is common to all muscles. When the chewing muscles are fatigued, the muscles that interact with them in the head and neck may work harder to guard them from further stress. Then these muscles, too, may become overworked and fatigued and trigger points may form in them as well.

Muscle fatigue and muscle guarding, alone or in combination, can eventually produce acute attacks of what is known as *myofascial pain dysfunction* syndrome, or *MPD*. The term *myofascial* refers to the muscle fibers themselves and to the fibrous connective tissue, or *fascia*, that surrounds them and binds them together. Myofascial pain can occur in any of several areas, depending on which muscles and trigger points are involved. The pain may be a headache, an earache, an ache in one or more teeth, an ache in the neck, even an ache in the shoulders or upper back—or several together.

Most patients with TMJ disorders suffer from myofascial pain to one extent or another. The basic cause can be malocclusion of the teeth, as described here, but it may have any of several other causes. And remember that the causes are more often multiple than single.

Malocclusion may also affect one or both of the TMJs themselves. The effect may be direct, if the malocclusion changes the position of the jaw enough to affect the placement of either condyle (see Figures 1 through 3). If the condyle is pushed too far backward and upward, for example, it is likely to exert heavy repeated pressure against the bone of the articular fossa every time the jaw closes in chewing. This is called *loading* the joint, and it produces *microtrauma* ("little injury") to the soft tissues. (Basketball players suffer this kind of joint loading in their knees from all the jumping and twisting they do.)

Repeated microtrauma irritates and inflames the tissues, especially the sensitive retrodiscal tissue and the capsule lining, the synovium. The various kinds of inflammation that occur in the joint, in fact, take their names from these tissues: *capsulitis* (*synovitis*) and *retrodiscitis*.

The pressure may also force the articular disk farther forward than it should be. This *anterior displacement* can have very serious consequences that are explained later in the chapter.

Finally, the effect of malocclusion on the TMJ may be exercised indirectly, through the supporting muscles. As already noted, an unbalanced bite can unbalance the muscles. The unbalanced muscles can in turn alter the position of either of the condyles or lead to displacement of its disk.

• Stress and the TMJ

Psychological stress can be defined as the response of the central nervous system to a powerful, disturbing stimulus from the environment. The term is often used in a negative way, to describe tension caused by the trials and tribulations of living. But stress doesn't have to be painful. Good news and pleasant changes can be stressful as well.

People respond to stress in many different ways. Here the focus is on one specific physical response—a response that has a profound effect on the TMJ and is directly related to several of its disorders: spontaneous clenching or grinding of the teeth.

Some people only clench. Some only grind. Some do both. Some clench or grind occasionally; some do so most or all of the time. Many are unaware of the habit and may even clench or grind in their sleep. Those who grind their teeth at night are an especial burden to those within earshot.

Clenching and grinding are hard on the teeth and should be discouraged, to the extent they can be consciously controlled. The healthy resting position for the mouth is with the lips closed, the tongue pressed lightly against the roof of the mouth, and the jaw slightly open. You shouldn't put any pressure on your teeth except when chewing and swallowing.

But damage to the teeth is only part of the problem, and not the worst part. For one thing, habitual clenching and grinding fatigue the chewing muscles. This fatigue, like that from maloccusion, can produce trigger points and MPD. Furthermore, grinding the teeth wears them down and can create malocclusion.

But the most serious damage, in terms of long-range consequences, occurs in the TMJ. You may recall the discussion in Chapter 2 of the superior belly of the lateral pterygoid muscle on each side of the jaw (see Figures 6 and 7). It attaches to the front of the condyle and the articular disk. It contracts only when the mandible closes and apparently stabilizes the "cushion" of the disk in the correct position as the condyle moves backward.

When food is being chewed, the muscle exerts just enough pressure to hold the disk in its proper place. But when the mandible closes, hard, on nothing, as when grinding the teeth, it exerts too strong a pressure—the joint becomes "loaded." Over a period of time the disk tends to be squeezed forward between the bones, rather like a watermelon seed squeezed between the fingers.

Eventually the disk is squeezed forward so far that it is no longer on top of the condyle. The retrodiscal tissue that connects it to the back of the capsule becomes stretched or even torn and can no longer hold it where it belongs. This is called *anterior disk displacement*, or *internal derangement*. In the process, the sensitive retrodiscal tissue may become inflamed and sore—the retrodiscitis mentioned before. Moreover, as the disk migrates forward, it can "escape" the condyle, producing the symptom known as *clicking*.

Figure 13 shows how clicking works: When the jaw is closed, the "escaped" disk is no longer on top of the condyle, but in front of it. As the jaw opens, the condyle translates forward and rides over the thick rear section of the disk. It then lands (or *reduces*) on the thin center section, and produces a noticeable click or pop. It remains on the thinner center until the jaw begins to close again. Then, at a certain point, it rides back over the thicker ridge and off the disk again. The result is a second click or pop. This condition is known formally as *internal derangement with reduction*.

Disk derangement serious enough to produce clicking is fairly common. Studies have found it to occur in at least 5 percent—one in twenty—of teenagers, and the percentage increases (as you might expect) with age. A dentist can measure the severity of the problem by *when* the clicking occurs in the chewing cycle. If the opening click is *early* and the closing click is *late*, the damage is less serious—the disk hasn't migrated very far forward. But if the opening click is *late* and the closing click *early*, the disk has migrated quite far and the chances of "recapturing" it are much lower.

Clicking may not be painful. If it's not, and if there are no other symptoms, it may not require treatment. Sometimes it goes away by itself. But if it continues and grows more severe, other troubles may follow.

For instance, the disk may continue migrating forward, and a most alarming symptom can appear. The condyle

Figure 13. Anterior disk displacement, with reduction.

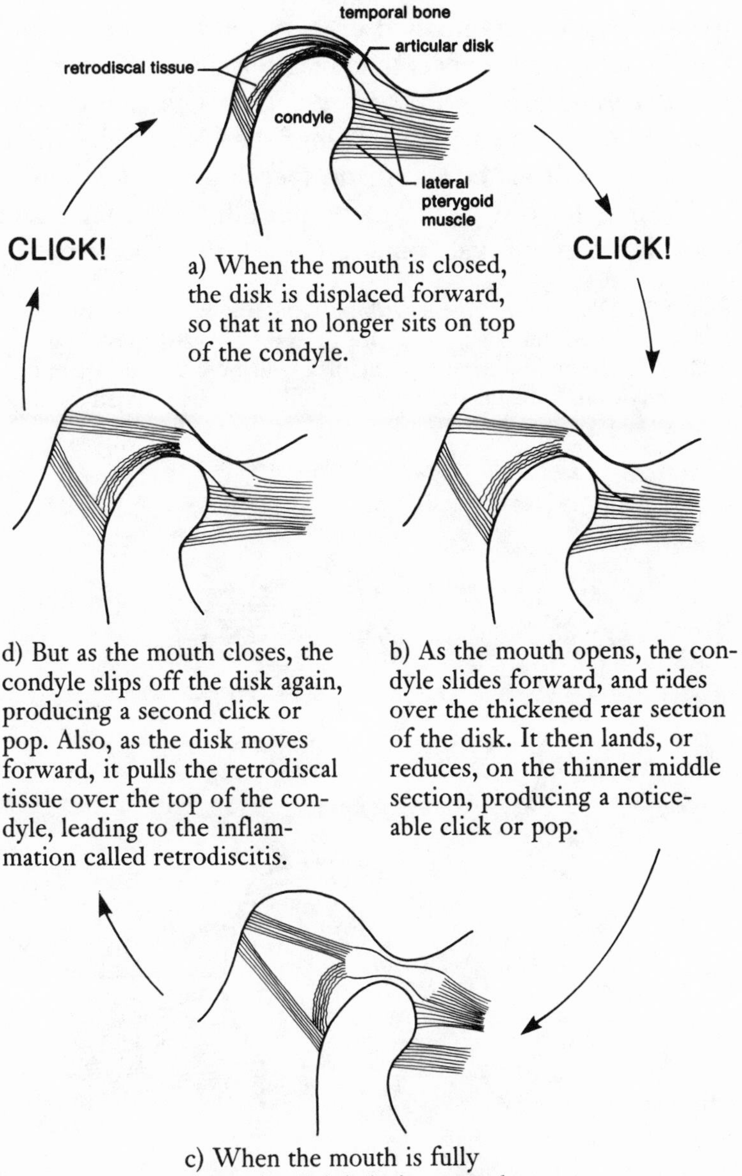

a) When the mouth is closed, the disk is displaced forward, so that it no longer sits on top of the condyle.

b) As the mouth opens, the condyle slides forward, and rides over the thickened rear section of the disk. It then lands, or reduces, on the thinner middle section, producing a noticeable click or pop.

c) When the mouth is fully open, the disk is in its normal position on top of the condyle.

d) But as the mouth closes, the condyle slips off the disk again, producing a second click or pop. Also, as the disk moves forward, it pulls the retrodiscal tissue over the top of the condyle, leading to the inflammation called retrodiscitis.

will no longer reduce on the disk (Figure 14). Instead, as the condyle translates forward, the disk rolls or folds up in front of it and gets mashed up between the condyle and the side of the eminence. The result: *closed locking* or, *internal derangement without reduction.* The jaw simply won't open past that point. Even if there's no pain (there usually is), normal chewing and speech are impossible.

At first, locking tends to be periodic—it comes and goes. But the intervals between attacks are likely to be-

Figure 14. Disk displacement without reduction. a) When the mouth is closed, the disk is displaced too far forward to be "captured." b) As the mouth opens, the disk rolls or folds up in front of the condyle, and prevents full opening. This is called closed locking.

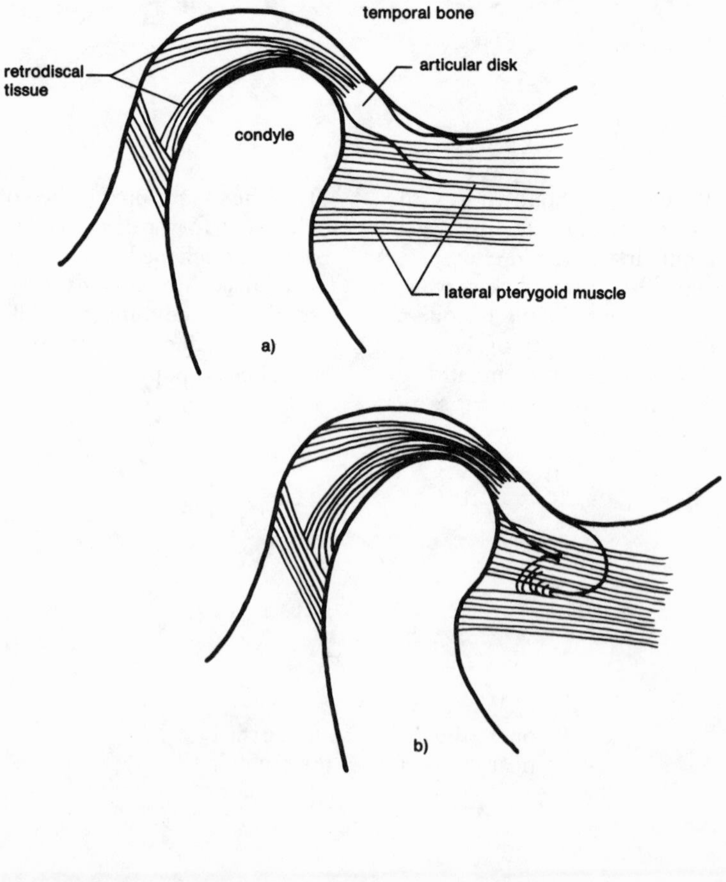

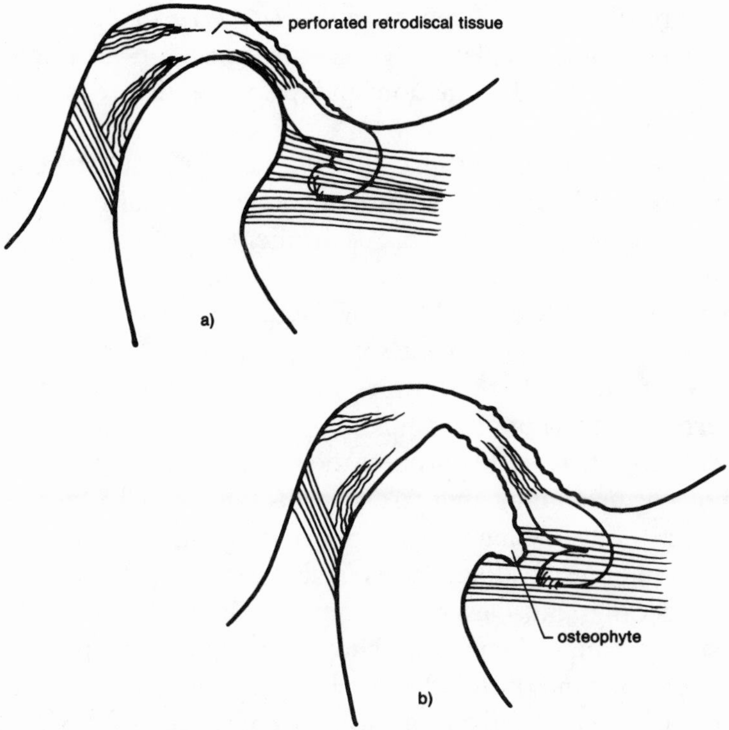

Figure 15. Disk damage and osteoarthritis. a) The displaced disk and stretched retrodiscal tissue eventually may become torn or worn through ("perforated"). Then, as the protection of the disk is lost, the bones themselves become damaged, a condition called osteoarthritis. b) The bearing surfaces become worn and rough, and bony spurs called osteophytes may develop on the condyle. The shape of the condyle changes, from a rounded knob to a flattened anvil.

come shorter and shorter, and the condition may eventually become permanent. Furthermore, if severe clicking and locking, or rather the derangement that causes them, is left unattended, friction on the disk and retrodiscal tissue may wear them through (*perforate* them) or even destroy them (Figure 15).

Worse, the unprotected surfaces of the bones can become worn and damaged as they rub against each other.

The result is bone degeneration, or *osteoarthritis*. Clicking and locking are replaced by a grating sensation called *crepitus*. Severe inflammation and pain are then virtually certain.

The only consolation is that the painful acute stage of osteoarthritis usually comes to an end over a period of six to eighteen months or so. A chronic "burned-out" stage follows. X-rays reveal that the bone surfaces have become flattened and harder. They rub together without pain or restriction of movement, although crepitus continues. This stage may last indefinitely or may be periodically interrupted by acute flare-ups.

At any stage in this process the muscles may become involved, producing myofascial pain. This can happen in several ways. Clenching and grinding may fatigue the chewing muscles themselves, making them stiff and sore. Then other muscles may begin guarding to reduce the pain and may themselves become fatigued and painful. The same kind of muscle guarding may result if an articular disk becomes displaced and the soft tissue of the joint becomes inflamed. Furthermore, trigger points may form in any of these fatigued muscles, referring pain to other parts of the body.

Clenching and grinding the teeth may have other adverse effects. We know, for example, that TMJ disorders appear to result from malocclusion and that clenching and grinding the teeth eventually wear them down. The result can be malocclusion severe enough to cause troubles in the joint or its muscles.

Pain is, of course, a major source of psychological stress. And the pain produced by TMJ disorders—either myofascial pain or inflammation of the joint itself—may contribute to the stress that led to the problem in the first place. Remember that both causes and effects are complex—and interrelated.

Clenching and grinding the teeth are very hard habits to break. Attempts at conscious control are likely to be unavailing, since very often the patient is not aware of the habit and continues even during sleep. Treatment must often be directed at the real cause, through either psychological therapy or behavior modification.

You may find it helpful at this point to review Figure 16, which shows the usual course of TMJ disorders related to each of these two major factors and the interaction that often occurs between them.

Figure 16. The course of TMJ disorders related to malocclusion and to grinding and clenching, and the interrelationship between them.

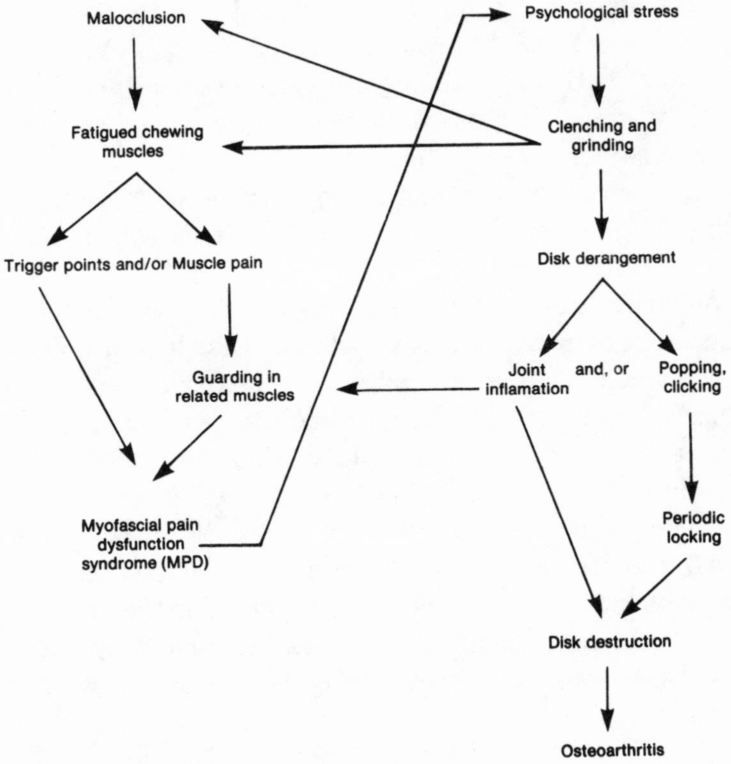

• Bad Postural Habits

Some bad habits you *can* do something about, either on your own or with the help of a physical therapist: habits of posture, particularly of the head and neck. Although they don't usually cause TMJ disorders all by themselves, they certainly aggravate the problems.

Undoubtedly as a child you were commanded to stand and sit up straight. There's a good reason. Your head weighs 12 or 13 pounds, and carrying it around all your waking hours is a considerable burden for your muscles—especially if it is not centered on your neck bones, the *cervical spine.* If you habitually carry your head too far forward, too far back, or too far to either side, the weight puts undesirable strain on the back and neck muscles, and they can then easily become fatigued. Not only can they become stiff and sore themselves, but through trigger points and muscle guarding may also produce pain elsewhere—including the head.

The postural habit that most often causes trouble for the TMJ is the forward-positioned head. The head is thrust forward and the chin tilted up (Figure 17) in what is sometimes called "bird-watcher's posture," because it is characteristic of people using binoculars. It is also common among people who are near-sighted and thrust their heads forward to read. People who work at computer terminals are likewise susceptible, especially if they have to strain forward to see the monitor clearly.

This habit can also result, unfortunately, from vanity. In our society, a receding chin is not considered attractive, for either men or women. A "weak chin" is even considered to betray a defect in character. So, some people who have a naturally small mandible tend to thrust it forward to compensate.

In any event, this forward position puts undesirable

pressure on the neck and back muscles, with the risk of fatigue. It also puts a strain on the TMJ, risking inflammation of the soft tissues.

Tipping the head sharply back can produce rather similar difficulties. If you have ever performed a task like painting a ceiling, which compels you to look and reach overhead for an extended period, you probably know how easy it is to get a stiff neck in the process. Serious muscle problems can result for those who habitually assume this unnatural posture.

When using the phone, many people cock their heads

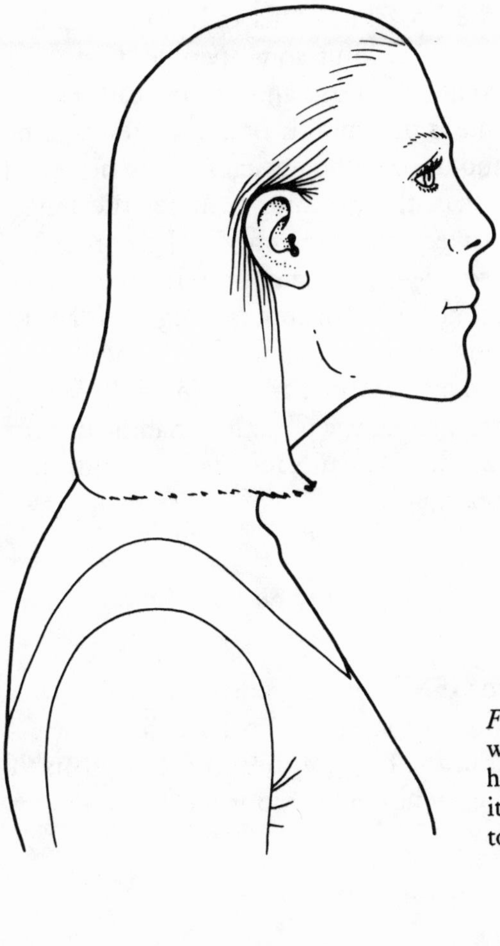

Figure 17. The forward-positioned head, a harmful postural habit that often contributes to TMJ disorders.

to one side and tuck the instrument between cheek and shoulder in order to leave both hands free. Those who do so habitually and for long periods of time may be in for serious problems with their neck muscles—and also with related muscles in their backs and heads. Perhaps because I practice in New York, where there are many musicians, I have an unusual number of patients who are violinists and who spend many hours a day with the instrument held between jaw and collarbone.

A couple of habits that can't exactly be called postural are closely related. I noted earlier, for example, that the most healthy resting position for the mouth is with the jaw slightly open and the lips shut. This of course requires breathing through the nose. But some people do not, or cannot, breathe through the nose and are instead *mouth-breathers*. The trouble is that mouth-breathing tends to be rapid and shallow and utilizes the muscles of the neck and upper chest rather than the diaphragm under the lungs. Fatigue in these muscles can aggravate TMJ disorders.

So can *tongue-thrusting*—habitually pressing the tongue hard against the front teeth or protruding it forward through the lips. This causes the main muscles activating the tongue to become overworked and fatigued. In fact, it can be said without too much exaggeration that the unnecessary tension of *any* muscle can cause fatigue, with potentially harmful consequences.

• Trauma

The basic causes for TMJ disorders discussed so far—malocclusion, response to stress, postural habits—originate essentially within the body, either in the TMJ itself or nearby. But one common and important cause comes from outside: mechanical injury, known technically as *trauma.* In our mobile society, the most common source of trauma is automobile accidents.

Collisions result in two main types of injuries. The first type is produced by a direct blow to the jaw and is usually the result of a front-end or side collision. The second is indirect (or *whiplash*) injury resulting from a rear-end collision.

If you're in a front-end or side collision, especially if you're not wearing a seatbelt, you're quite likely to strike your face on the dashboard or steering wheel, against one of the doors, or against the front seat if you're riding in back. If the blow is to the lower part of your face, your lower jaw is likely to be shoved suddenly and sharply backward. (The same thing can happen if you suffer a fall or are struck on the jaw.)

Even if you're lucky enough not to fracture the jawbone, the capsule of one or both joints will receive a serious wrench. This can irritate the synovial lining of the capsule, causing the inflammation called capsulitis or synovitis. Moreover, one or both of the condyles may be driven backward into the sensitive retrodiscal tissue, causing retrodiscitis.

Capsulitis and retrodiscitis are not only painful in themselves, they can also produce myofascial pain, muscle guarding, trigger points, and referred pain. A common symptom in these cases is a severe recurrent headache that appears days, weeks, even months after the accident and thus seems unrelated to it.

In this context another complication can be very serious, especially if it isn't treated right away. When injury causes bleeding in the retrodiscal tissue (which is well supplied with blood vessels), *ankylosis,* or permanent stiffening, may result. Hard, fibrous tissue forms in the joint, severely restricting its range of movement. To put it even more simply, you can hardly get your mouth open. The only treatment is surgery.

When your jaw is struck directly, it's usually pretty obvious from bruises or contusions on the skin. But a whiplash injury from a rear-end collision isn't so obvious. Your head may not have hit anything, and there may be no visible damage at all. But the injury can be just as serious.

Whiplash is a good name for this two-stage process (Figure 18). When your car is struck from behind, the impact drives your seat and body forward, but inertia tends to keep your head where it was. So it "whips" backward on the flexible column of your neck. Then, when the impact ends, inertia works in the opposite direction. As your

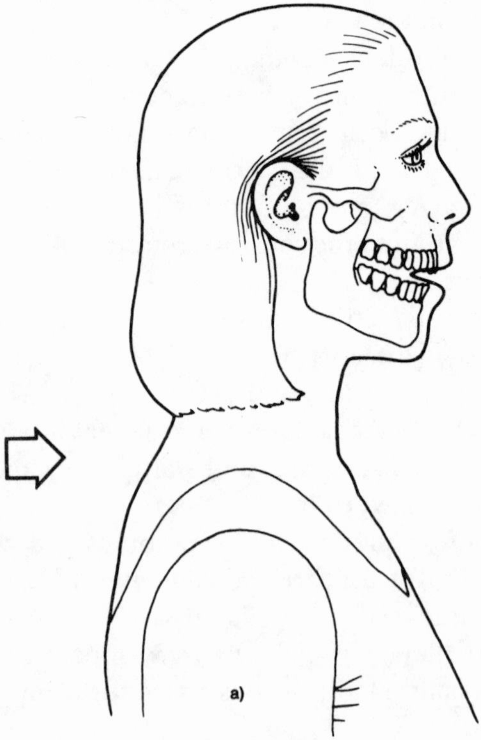

a)

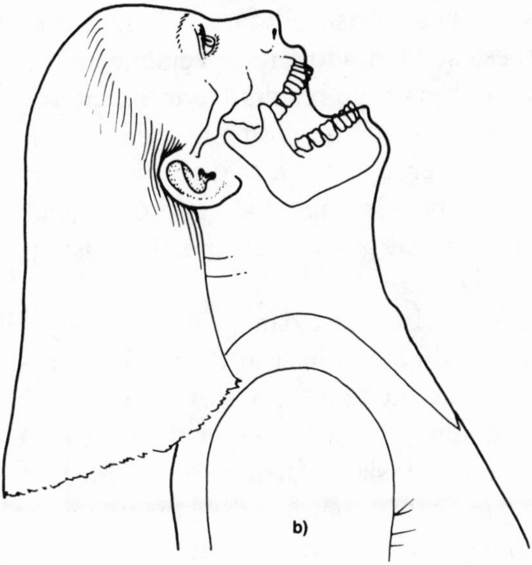

b)

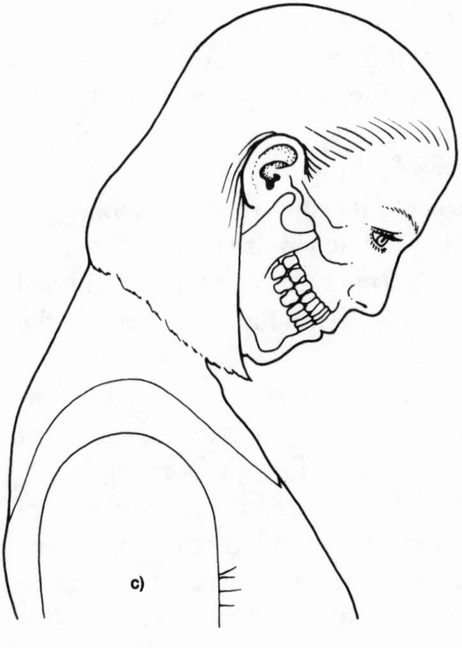

c)

Figure 18. Whiplash injury. a) When your car is struck from behind, your seat and body are suddenly thrust forward, but inertia tends to hold your head in place. b) As a result, your head is whipped backward on your neck, opening the jaws too wide, and straining the joint, and the head and neck muscles. c) As the car stops, your head lashes forward, snapping the jaws shut, and further straining the joint and the muscles.

car stops, your head "lashes" forward. Damage results from both these sudden, violent movements.

Much whiplash damage results from instinctive action of the neck muscles. At the moment of impact, in just a millisecond, they tense to protect the head from bobbing about uncontrollably. In the process, the muscles themselves may be strained or torn, eventually causing trigger points and MPD.

But the muscles also cause damage to the TMJs. When the cranium is "whipped" backward, the lighter, smaller mandible is held by the tense muscles under the chin and the jaw is suddenly opened far wider than usual. As a result, each condyle translates farther forward than normal. In really extreme cases, the mandible may be completely dislocated (or *luxated*) out of the joints.

Usually, though, the mandible becomes only partially dislocated, or *subluxated.* Serious harm may nonetheless be done. As each condyle is suddenly thrust forward, the articular disk may be squeezed so as to be partly or entirely in front of it. The disk itself may be perforated, or the retrodiscal tissue attached to the disk may be stretched or torn. Worse, the disk may "escape" the condyle, causing disk displacement or even locking.

After the head whips back, it lashes forward, tending to make the jaw close too hard. The result is rather like a direct blow. In one or both joints the condyle is rammed backward, stretching the capsule and further damaging the retrodiscal tissue.

Once again, symptoms may be delayed or may be temporarily masked by other injuries. An example is a recent patient of mine, a college student I'll call Dorothy Prior. She was driving down a main city avenue one winter evening, when her car was struck on the left rear side by another car pulling out of a side street. Her car was totaled; she not only got a whiplash injury but badly twisted her neck and back as well. No bones were broken, but she underwent a month of physical therapy to treat her wrenched muscles.

Two months after the accident, in early spring, she noticed clicking in the right side of her jaw. Shortly afterward, she began to suffer headaches and earaches on the same side. She didn't associate any of these symptoms with the accident, from which she thought she had completely recovered.

Through the spring and summer, her symptoms became gradually worse. By June she was having trouble opening her mouth and chewing. On the Fourth of July the pain reached a climax, and her face swelled up. She thought the problem might be her wisdom teeth and began what was to be a series of visits to different dentists. None of them found anything wrong with her teeth. One of them suspected a TMJ inflammation and provided conservative treatment to relieve it. After several months, however, she was still in pain. Her older sister, a nurse, then referred her to me.

When I examined her, Dorothy was suffering inflammation in the right joint—inflammation that was being prolonged and intensified by a displaced disk. Pain was also being referred to muscles in her face and head, accounting for the headaches and earaches. All these symptoms had their origins in the accident almost a year earlier. Treatment for the displacement gradually but surely relieved them.

• Open, Please—But Not Too Wide

Dramatic events like accidents aren't the only circumstances that can produce trauma in the TMJs. Trauma can result from overly wide jaw-opening of any kind. Some authorities maintain that the damage can be done voluntarily—by overenergetic yawning, say, or biting into a very thick sandwich. I have run into very few such cases in my own experience. But I have encountered several patients who have been injured by *involuntary* opening.

The first commandment in medicine is "Do no harm." I therefore regret to report that one cause of trauma from excessive opening is medical and dental treatment. In dentistry, it is likely to be a procedure requiring extensive and prolonged opening—such as the extraction of a deeply rooted wisdom tooth. In medical treatment, it is surgery under general anesthesia. The second of these two can be especially damaging.

The usual procedure for general anesthesia is to render the patient unconscious, then to administer oxygen and anesthetic gases through a tube down the throat—a process called *intubation*. The mouth must be held open quite wide, and since the relaxed, unfeeling muscles offer no resistance, it's not hard to overdo the procedure. Severe inflammation, and sometimes disk displacement as well, can result.

This problem doesn't occur often, but it is a recognized complication of surgery, and a recent patient of mine, Irene Thorpe, suffered from it. She had undergone abdominal surgery, and when she woke up she could hardly open her mouth. The cause was trauma from intubation during her operation, which had displaced the disks in both joints. Over time the range of movement improved only a little, and she continued to suffer soreness in her jaw, then severe earaches. Ordinary treatment proved ineffective, and TMJ surgery was eventually required.

I should mention in passing one other possible ill effect from medical treatment. This one involves not opening the mouth too wide but closing it too tight.

Until rather recently it was common to treat neck and

back injuries with *traction,* a process by which the skull was literally pulled away from the neck and back bones in order to reduce pressure on the joints between them. The usual mechanism for this purpose was a sling that was placed under the chin and attached to pulleys and weights so as to exert strong, steady pressure. Unfortunately, the sling also forced the jaw to clamp shut, often producing microtrauma and joint inflammation in the process.

Lately, physicians and physical therapists have become more sensitive to this problem and have devised slings that do not put pressure on the chin. But inflammation resulting from traction still turns up from time to time.

• What Else Could It Be?

Beware of anybody—your physician, your dentist, your best friend, whoever—who hears about your aches and pains and says right off, "You have a TMJ problem." There are other diseases, lots of them, that can produce the same symptoms. Headaches, in particular, have literally hundreds of causes. Indeed, diagnosing a malady as a TMJ disorder, when the true cause is something else, may be dangerous as well as useless.

The case of a patient at our clinic illustrates the potential danger. Thirty-five-year-old Nancy Worth was referred to us by a dentist who had been treating her over a period of four months for what he thought was a TMJ disorder. Her condition wasn't improving, and he had come to doubt his diagnosis. She suffered intermittent pain and had a slight swelling in front of her left ear. Treatment wasn't helping.

About six months before, when she first noticed the problem, she had been examined by an internist and an ear-nose-throat specialist. At that time no sign of disease or other abnormality was found. She had then gone to the dentist, who found the muscular pain—MPD—typical of a TMJ disorder. He began a conservative course of treatment designed primarily to relieve the pain. It didn't work. Rather than proceeding further, he consulted us.

In addition to examining Mrs. Worth for a TMJ disorder we gave her other tests. In particular, we were troubled by the swelling in front of her ear. Our radiologist suggested that the usual X-rays be supplemented with the sophisticated scanning procedure known as *computed tomography* (*CT*). It not only provides a complete cross-section view of the head but is also sensitive enough to reveal details of soft tissue as well as bone.

In this case, CT revealed a tumor next to the left TMJ. When it was surgically removed, it proved to be a cancer of the parotid gland, a salivary gland located close to the TMJ. Fortunately, it appears to have been caught in time. The surgery was successful, and there has been no sign of cancer, there or elsewhere, since.

Cancer is only one of the serious ills that must be ruled out in the process of *differential diagnosis*, a process I'll describe more fully in the next chapter. It lies far beyond the scope of this book to list all the things that aren't really TMJ disorders yet produce similar symptoms. I'll mention only a couple.

Perhaps the most misleading of the TMJ "lookalikes" is *trigeminal neuralgia*, sometimes called by its French name, *tic douloureux*. This is a disorder of the trigeminal nerve—the "three-branched" nerve that registers sensations from the TMJ and its surrounding structures. But trigeminal neuralgia is fundamentally different from such TMJ disorders as MPD or capsulitis. In TMJ disorders, pain originates in the chewing muscles or in the joint. In trigeminal neuralgia, the nerve itself is diseased. It seldom occurs in people under thirty-five, and its causes are not known.

The pain of trigeminal neuralgia is also distinctive: a sharp, occasional shooting pain rather than the persistent ache typical of TMJ disorders. Differential diagnosis can nevertheless be difficult. Once more, I cannot overemphasize the importance of communication and collaboration between specialists in different fields—in this case, dentist and neurologist. If the patient is middle-aged or older and if the pain stabs rather than aches, trigeminal neuralgia should be suspected, and he or she should be referred for neurological examination.

Another common TMJ lookalike disorder, especially among older patients, is *rheumatoid arthritis*, a mystery disease that produces inflammation and eventual breakdown of the joints. Nobody knows what causes it, or how to cure it, or why more women than men suffer from it.

Rheumatoid arthritis is characterized by chronic stiffness and pain, especially first thing in the morning, before the joints are exercised. The TMJ can be one of the joints affected, and the main symptom is inflammation of the capsule lining—synovitis—just like the synovitis in other TMJ disorders.

In the course of time, the disease may attack the structures of the joint itself. It can "eat up" the cartilage protecting the bone surfaces and the bone material itself (in the TMJ it tends to attack the condyle). This condition is both painful and severely debilitating. One possible result is an *open bite*, in which the front teeth no longer come together when the jaw is closed. Finally, ankylosis may set in. Hard, fibrous tissue forms in what is left of the joint, further limiting its movement.

Rheumatoid arthritis is one of a family of arthritic diseases that produce symptoms like those of TMJ disorders.

Usually they are not hard to differentiate from myofascial pain or disk dislocation. Arthritic disease almost never appears in the TMJs alone but is found in other joints as well, particularly those in the hands. As one authority puts it, "Hands are the calling card of the arthritic." Furthermore, such a disease usually produces changes in the blood that can be identified in standard tests.

Nevertheless, some of the same treatments used for TMJ disorders can at times be helpful to arthritis patients. For example, the same anti-inflammatory medications are used for both conditions. I'll describe these in Chapter 5.

FOUR

Going for Help

THE DIAGNOSIS OF TMJ DISORDERS

With increasing frequency over about three years, Roberta Steele suffered headaches in her temples and at the base of her skull. She didn't know what caused them. Like most of us, she took a couple of aspirin, and after several hours the discomfort went away.

But gradually the headaches got worse and worse. Then she developed another symptom, a noticeable clicking whenever she opened and closed her jaw. When she began to suffer pain in front of her left ear, she went to her dentist, thinking she might have a toothache. He believed a malocclusion was causing her problems, and selectively ground some of her teeth to give her a more even bite.

This didn't help, and she didn't know where to turn next. A friend gave her the name of an oral surgeon associated with our clinic at Mount Sinai. He told her that she had a TMJ disorder and that she might need surgery. But first he sent her to us, to confirm the diagnosis and to see if more conservative treatment would suffice.

We agreed with his diagnosis and concluded that conservative, nonsurgical treatment was indeed appropriate.

The headaches, the clicking, and the pain in the joint all derived from a forward dislocation of the articular disk, of the kind described in Chapter 3. The course of treatment we provided satisfactorily relieved her symptoms. Mrs. Steele was almost as glad to learn the nature of the disorder as to be freed of pain. "It was a miracle," she told me, "to find anyone who knew what the problem was. I thought I was going crazy."

• Where to Start

If you have a disorder involving the TMJs, how do you go about getting help? Well, you won't necessarily start out with someone who concentrates in that area; in fact, like Mrs. Steele, you probably won't.

At first you may not know or suspect that you have a TMJ problem at all. TMJ disorders are painful pretenders that often produce symptoms elsewhere—and the same symptoms can also result from other ailments. In fact, it is absolutely essential to separate and identify the true source of the symptoms and to examine and rule out any others. This process is called *differential diagnosis* and, as I have already noted, it often requires the pooled knowledge of experts in several fields.

If your main symptom is a chronic headache, you will probably first consult your general practitioner or internist, or possibly a neurologist. There are many organic causes of headaches; they should be considered and ruled out before you jump to the conclusion that a TMJ disorder is involved. Likewise, if you have a recurrent earache, you may consult an ear-nose-throat specialist to rule out the infections and other ailments that often cause this symptom. If you have persistent pain in the neck or upper back, you might see an orthopedist, who may find a postural problem or a spine or muscle disorder that doesn't involve the TMJ at all. And, if the symptom is pain in the teeth or the jaw itself, you will probably consult a dentist—but you should recognize that he or she may have to refer you to someone else if TMJ treatment is required.

If the physician or dentist cannot clearly establish the cause of your problem after diagnostic procedures, *then* you should request a referral for a TMJ examination. This is especially true if your symptoms include one or more of these:

- *Pain when opening or closing the jaw.* The entire movement may be painful, or it may be restricted. You may not be able to open beyond a certain point without pain, or muscle guarding may make complete opening difficult if not impossible.
- *Inability to open the mouth straight.* You may be able to see this in a mirror. If your jaw slips noticeably to one side as you open it, the cause may be a disorder in one of the TMJs.
- *Tenderness of the TMJ*, on either side or on both sides. The joint is located directly in front of the ear. You can feel it easily by lightly pressing your fingertips on this area, then opening and closing your mouth. If it hurts to do this, the joint may be inflamed.
- *Pain or tenderness in any of the chewing muscles*, especially those used to close the jaw. You can easily feel the thick masseter muscle, which extends diagonally from the angle of the jaw to the cheekbone, and the fan-shaped temporalis muscle on the temple, above and in front of the ear. The pterygoid muscles are not accessible this way, but you can assess their condition by a few *resistance tests.*

For instance, with the mouth partly open, press three fingers against the lower front teeth—firmly but not hard—and then close the jaw against this resistance. Likewise, with the jaw closed, press a fist against your chin and open against the resistance. Finally, press an open palm against each side of the lower jaw in turn and move the jaw sideways against the resistance. If any of these tests cause noticeable pain, one or more of the muscles may be fatigued and inflamed.

- *Noticeable clicking or popping* when opening or closing the mouth, or both. By itself, with none of the other symptoms present, this is not necessarily evidence of a serious TMJ disorder. Nevertheless, it is a classic symptom of disk derangement.

I am *not* recommending do-it-yourself diagnosis. Even if you find that you have some of these symptoms, a great deal more information is required and must be analyzed by expert professionals. But I do consider such symptoms enough to warrant a thorough TMJ examination.

Even if your physician or dentist determines that your problem is something else and undertakes treatment, the possibility of TMJ involvement should not be dismissed or forgotten. This is especially true if the treatment isn't effective. The headache, the earache, the pain in the neck or shoulder keeps coming back or even gets worse, and the practitioner can offer no good reason to explain it. It is time to request a referral for a TMJ examination.

• Finding an Expert

Your regular dentist may or may not be prepared to diagnose and treat TMJ disorders. The TMJ is indeed an area best understood by dentists, but treating it is not yet a recognized specialty, like oral surgery or orthodontics. It has no body of established standards. At many dental schools, it is not even taught as a separate topic.

Properly treating TMJ disorders nevertheless requires a good deal of special training. It can't be picked up just by reading the technical literature or by taking a short course. And the training must be reinforced by experience; it must be a regular part of the dentist's practice. How are you to judge whether your dentist has this kind of expertise?

You can perhaps judge in part by how thoroughly you are examined, something I'll discuss in more detail shortly. But even before the examination starts you don't have to be shy about asking what your dentist's training has been in the field, whether TMJ treatment is a regular part of his or her practice, and approximately how many such patients are treated in a year. If you have any doubts, you can at least seek a second opinion. You should certainly do so if the recommended treatment is extensive or drastic—surgery, say, or heavy dental reconstruction.

If you have to seek out a TMJ expert on your own, there are several sources for the names of practitioners who are active in the field. The American Dental Association, for example, is made up of state and local dental societies. The address and phone number of the one closest to you will be in your local phone book (listed as Dental Society, followed by the state or district) and may be able to give you names of dentists in your area who offer TMJ treatment. Caution: a dental society lists all its members who claim to be TMJ practitioners; it has no way of evaluating them.

Your local dental society may also be able to tell you whether members in your area have established a study group on TMJ disorders. I belong to such a group in New York, and its members include many of the active practitioners in the city.

Dentists with a special interest in TMJ disorders may belong to other professional associations as well, including the following:

- American Equilibration Society
- American Academy of Craniomandibular Disorders (AACD)
- Academy of Head, Neck and Facial Pain and Temporomandibular Joint Orthopedics

These organizations, whose addresses appear in the Appendix, will supply you the names of their members.

Another possible source of information is a comprehensive medical center or a university dental school. Such an institution—like Mount Sinai in New York—may actually have a special TMJ clinic. Even if it doesn't, it may be able to supply the names of dentists to whom it refers patients. Even if the institution itself is not in your immediate vicinity, it may know of someone who is.

You may not have to go through any of this. Your physician or dentist may refer you to a specific practitioner. This can have several advantages, especially if your own physician or dentist has collaborated with the TMJ practitioner in the past. Since TMJ disorders often require a multidisciplinary attack, if there's already a working relationship between someone who regularly treats you and the person who is examining you for a TMJ problem, you may be better off.

• The TMJ Examination

Now, let's suppose you've been examined for other possible causes of your symptoms, and all have been ruled out. You have found a dentist or clinic you consider qualified to diagnose and treat TMJ disorders. What kind of examination should you expect?

Answer: a thorough one. The goal is a reliable differential diagnosis. Before any treatment is begun, three questions must be answered:

• Is it certain that the problem is a TMJ disorder and not something else?

• What kind of TMJ disorder is it? Is it primarily a muscle problem? A disk-displacement problem? A trauma problem? A combination?

• Is it only a TMJ problem, or are other factors—such as disease, or injury in other parts of the body—also involved?

The first step should be a complete medical history and a history of your symptoms, including whatever previous examination and treatment you have had. The examiner may get this information from you orally or may give you a form to fill out. He or she may ask your permission to consult those who have treated you earlier—it is in fact desirable that any new practitioner do so.

• The Physical Exam

Next you will probably receive a physical examination. Don't be surprised if the examiner asks you to stand up and walk around. Postural problems, such as uneven gait, can cause pain in areas as far off as the neck and head. They can also contribute to the severity of TMJ disorders.

And don't be surprised if parts of your body other than your head are examined—particularly your neck, upper back, shoulders, and arms, which are often involved with TMJ problems. The examiner may even examine your hands; they can reveal whether arthritic disease is causing the problem or contributing to it.

You may be asked some rather personal questions about your life, and particularly about the amount of stress in it. You may be asked whether you are having any special problems at home or work, how soundly you sleep, and whether your appetite and digestion are healthy. Since stress is a major source of TMJ problems, this information is relevant.

If you haven't already been examined by a dentist, you may be given a dental examination, including standard dental X-rays, to make sure that your teeth and gums are healthy and that your pain doesn't come from something like an abscess or tooth decay.

Your occlusion—bite—will certainly be checked. Quite likely you will be asked to bite down on a thin sheet of colored paper or wax to show exactly how the upper and lower teeth meet. And, even during your first appointment, you may have molds made of your upper and lower teeth for diagnosis then and treatment later.

The examiner will subject you to a fair amount of palpation—pressing, poking, and prodding—outside and inside your mouth, all over your face and head, and along your neck, shoulders, and back. No mystery about this. He or she is checking for tightness and tenderness in the TMJs and the surrounding muscles and is looking for areas that either may be stiff or sore themselves or serve as trigger points for pain elsewhere.

The functioning of your muscles may also be checked with a series of *resistance tests* of the kind mentioned earlier in this chapter. If moving your jaw or head in a certain direction against resistance produces pain, that fact helps pinpoint the specific muscles involved.

Some practitioners use an *electromyograph* (*EMG*) machine for this purpose. It measures and records the electrical activity of individual muscles, and thus signals those that are working too hard, or going into spasm.

Your *range of movement* (*ROM*) will be checked. For example, how far can you open your mouth? The normal rule is that you should be able to insert three fingers of your hand between your upper and lower front teeth. If you can get in four, the jaw may be opening more than it should. It may easily become dislocated or inflamed. If you can't insert more than two fingers, or not even two, you have what's called *restricted* range of movement. Normal eating and speech are difficult if not impossible.

Even if you can open your mouth fully, can you open it straight? If your mandible deviates to one side as it descends, there may be a problem in the muscles or the joint on one side. You should also have free and painless movement in your jaw from side to side.

The range of movement of your head and neck will also be checked. In all these tests it is likely that both your *active* and *passive* ranges of movement (*AROM* and *PROM*) will be measured. Your active range of movement is the extent you can move your jaw, head, and neck by yourself; your passive range is the extent that the examiner can move them for you while you relax. Painful or restricted AROM suggests a muscle disorder; the same condition in PROM suggests a joint disorder such as inflammation. Of course, you may well suffer from both.

All these procedures give the joints and the chewing muscles something of a workout. As a result they may become temporarily more sore and sensitive than before the examination. Unfortunately, this can't be helped, but the condition is usually just temporary.

• Getting a Closer Look

A number of other tests will be devoted to finding out what's happening in each joint beneath the visible, palpable surface. For instance, a good deal can be learned from *listening,* especially if the disorder is a displaced articular disk. The examiner may listen for joint clicking through an ordinary medical stethoscope as you open and close your jaw. The timing and intensity of the clicking, as the condyle rides on and off the disk, help reveal the seriousness of the problem.

Nowadays the experience and intuition of the examiner may be supplemented by electronic amplification and computer analysis of the sound. A click of a certain duration and frequency, for instance, is strong evidence of a disk so far forward that locking is imminent.

A variety of other modern techniques is used to look beneath the surface. One that has recently come into use is *thermography*—("heat picture"). It provides a color-coded image of temperature variation along the side of the face, which can help locate areas of inflammation (relatively hot) or reduced circulation (relatively cool). But much more usual are various *imaging* techniques, and the most common of all are X-rays.

You can think of an X-ray itself as a beam of powerful, penetrating light, and the image on film as a negative shadow cast by this beam as it passes through various kinds of material. A more pronounced shadow will be cast by a dense material like bone than by soft tissue.

Ordinary dental X-rays are not sensitive enough to distinguish much more than bone. Similar ones are used to examine the TMJ, but mainly as a screening tool. They can show the approximate placement of the condyle in relation to the temporal bone when the jaw is opened and closed. They can also reveal bone disorders, such as degeneration from osteoarthritis. But they won't show the position of the articular disk or the condition of other soft tissues such as the joint capsule or the retrodiscal tissue.

Some dentists have a special X-ray machine that produces a *panoramic* image showing the whole arc of the jaws from ear to ear. It is often called a *Panorex* (the name of one particular brand). The patient stands or sits before the machine as the X-ray generator and the film, mounted on tracks, circle halfway around the head while the exposure is being made. Like ordinary X-rays, panorex is used chiefly as a screening device to reveal such problems as bone deformities, impacted teeth, fractures, and the like.

A more precise view of each joint is provided by a relatively sophisticated X-ray technique called *tomography* ("picture of a slice"), which requires bulky special equipment usually available only at a medical center or the office of a medical radiologist. The X-ray beam is focused, somewhat the way a light camera is focused, so that only one thin layer of the subject is sharp.

Tomograms are usually made in series, each one focused at a different level. Such a series provides quite a detailed assessment of the condyle and temporal bone, from which an experienced examiner can sometimes deduce where the disk is located. Still, tomograms don't tell much about the soft tissues.

The soft tissue that most often needs to be examined is the articular disk, and there are three imaging techniques used to get a look at it. Like tomography, they require relatively sophisticated and expensive machines; you won't find any of them in the dentist's office. Each has its own particular merits.

The method that's been in use the longest, *arthrography* ("picture of the joint"), is still the "gold standard" by which other methods are measured. A liquid dye opaque to X-rays is injected into the capsule of the joint. On film, the dye-filled cavity appears as a well-defined, very light area. An expert examiner can deduce from the particular shape of this area whether the nearby disk is displaced or damaged.

Arthrography has one big advantage over other imaging techniques: it can be viewed live—an enlarged, continuous view can be shown on a fluoroscope screen. It can reveal, in motion, how the position of the disk changes as the jaw opens and closes. The fluoroscope display can be recorded on videotape for later review. For some patients, the dye injection for arthrography causes temporary discomfort. This can usually be soothed with the application of ice as soon as the examination is over.

The second technique is *computerized tomography*, or *CT*—what used to be called a CAT scan. In Chapter 3, I mentioned its use in diagnosing an otherwise invisible cancer. CT produces only still images, but it is sensitive enough to reveal subtle details of both bone and soft tissue and provides a view of the disk.

The third imaging technique is called nuclear magnetic resonance (NMR) or magnetic resonance imaging (MRI). It produces still images of great sensitivity and has the advantage of not requiring radiation. It is not yet as widely available as the other two, but is becoming more and more popular for many medical applications.

Such advanced techniques are not necessary or appropriate in every case, but all three are immensely valuable diagnostic tools. There is nothing like them for looking under the surface to view conditions that otherwise might only be guessed at. Which one your examiner chooses is likely to depend upon the availability of equipment and—perhaps even more important—of skilled, experienced operators. Getting clear, reliable results from any of these methods is as much an art as a science.

• Special Studies

Just as another physician or dentist may refer you for a TMJ examination, the examiner may refer you in turn to other specialists, especially if there is any evidence that some other disorder is involved. These might include an internist, a neurologist, an ear-nose-throat specialist, an oral surgeon, or a rheumatologist (expert on arthritis).

The TMJ examiner might collaborate with one or more of these other specialists in arranging for procedures such as blood tests, to check for the special blood components that indicate an underlying disease like arthritis and to rule out infections that might produce TMJ "lookalike" symptoms.

• The TMJ Diagnosis

Once the examination is completed—a process that may require more than one appointment—the examiner will probably come up with a diagnosis. You may be told that there is no evidence, or not enough, to justify a diagnosis of a TMJ disorder. Fair enough. But if there are doubts in your mind and your symptoms can't be explained in any other way, you might well seek another opinion.

You should be far more cautious if you are given only a perfunctory examination and the examiner wants to plunge right in with treatment. Not every practitioner uses all the tools and procedures I've mentioned, and other experts may have done the necessary work to rule out other possible diagnoses. Nevertheless, at the very least, the TMJ examination should include the complete history and the basic physical examination described.

But let's suppose that you've had a thorough exam and have been diagnosed as having a TMJ disorder. Now treatment is recommended. Before going ahead, you should be given frank and detailed answers to three basic questions:

- *What's the matter?* What specific type of TMJ disorder is present? Or, if that can't be established for certain, what is the most likely possibility? Myofascial pain? Disk dislocation? Joint inflammation? A combination?

• *What's to be done?* What course of treatment is proposed? How many steps are involved, and how long are they likely to take? What is treatment likely to cost—not just in money, but also in time, energy, discomfort?

• *What can be achieved?* What is the aim of the treatment? Complete cure? (That may not be realistic or practical.) Alleviation of pain? Reaching a particular level of activity or comfort? And what are the chances of success—or failure?

The TMJ practitioner may not be able to provide precise, simple answers to all these questions but should give you at least a range of the possibilities and alternatives. If he or she is vague about these matters or seems to be "winging it," be cautious. There is nothing wrong with seeking a second opinion.

FIVE

Finding Relief

BASIC TMJ TREATMENT

Melissa Sontag, a woman in her early thirties, came to me a few weeks after suffering a rather unusual injury. She had been playing in a friendly office softball game when a wild throw by one of her teammates caught her square on the right side of her jaw. The impact was so great, she reported, that the ball had left the pattern of its stitching in bruises on her face.

She had spent three weeks in great pain, barely able to open her mouth. X-rays showed no broken bones, and the main therapy her physician prescribed was the application of ice packs to reduce pain and swelling.

I had treated a friend of hers following an automobile accident, so when Ms. Sontag still couldn't open her mouth comfortably after almost a month, she thought of me. When I examined her, I concluded that she was suffering from severe inflammation in the right joint. When the ball had struck her on the jaw, the nearby condyle had apparently been driven hard into the fossa, inflaming the joint capsule (capsulitis) and the retrodiscal tissue (retrodiscitis).

I started a course of basic treatment that is effective for most TMJ patients, whatever the cause of their disorder. Known as *phase-one* treatment, its principal goal is the alleviation of symptoms—in this instance the pain of inflammation.

Phase-one treatment is deliberately conservative. Its procedures are all *reversible:* nothing is done that can't be undone later. (Phase-two treatment is made up largely of procedures that are *irreversible;* I describe these in Chapter 8.) Much phase-one treatment wasn't developed specifically for TMJ disorders. Rather, it consists of tried-and-true techniques used by physicians, chiropractors, osteopaths, and physical therapists to relieve all kinds of muscle and joint pain, from a sprained ankle to tennis elbow.

• Cold and Heat Therapy

I began Melissa Sontag's treatment with the cold therapy already prescribed by her physician. Its usual form is the application of ice for periods of no more than twenty minutes in any hour (anything longer than that can do serious damage to the skin). For inflamed joints, chilling generally seems to be the most effective temporary remedy.

Some patients, though, respond better with heat—usually the method of choice when the pain comes from muscle spasm rather than joint inflammation. (I discuss various cold and heat treatments in greater detail in Chapter 6, pages xx-xx.)

• "Walking-Cane" Therapies

I also had Ms. Sontag undertake what I call "walking-cane" therapies. When you sprain an ankle, you can lean on a cane or crutch to avoid putting unnecessary weight on it. Likewise, there are various ways to avoid putting unnecessary pressure on an inflamed TMJ. The first and most obvious is to limit its movement. I tell patients to open their lower jaws only so far as they feel no pain, and to avoid wide opening of any sort. If they feel a yawn coming on, they should restrict it by pressing a fist under the chin.

Just as the jaw shouldn't open too wide, it shouldn't close too hard. This usually requires a temporary change to a soft diet. I don't mean you have to switch entirely to liquids and baby food. That extreme a diet is necessary only for those few who can hardly open their mouths at all. Most patients just need to avoid foods like raw vegetables, nuts, hard rolls, and chewy meat such as steak. And, needless to say, chewing gum is out.

Instead, you can substitute main dishes such as casseroles and hashes made with chopped or minced meat and fish. Pasta and noodle dishes are also easy on the jaws, and so, of course, are soups. Cooked vegetables and fruits can be substituted for raw and supplemented with juices. For dessert, puddings, custards, and ice cream give little or no work to the joints or their surrounding muscles. As a demonstration of what can be accomplished within these limits, one enterprising author has written and published a *Non-Chew Cookbook*. Information on ordering it is included in the Appendix.

Incidentally, a soft diet isn't going to be much help if you don't stick to it. Inflammation takes a while to subside—usually at least a few weeks, and certainly not just a few days.

Some practitioners believe that TMJ patients benefit not only from a soft diet but also from supplements of extra vitamins. I don't know of any scientific evidence that vitamins specifically relieve muscular pain or joint inflammation. But without question, a nutritious, balanced diet is important, especially during recovery from an ailment. Also, a soft diet, with its limits on raw fruits and vegetables, will tend to be less rich in certain vitamins, especially vitamins A and C and some of the B complex. So, although I myself don't believe that extra vitamins are essential, it is perfectly reasonable to include them in a course of treatment.

There is, however, one temporary dietary change that I often do recommend: I advise patients in pain to cut down on, or even eliminate, their intake of caffeine. Caffeine is a stimulant to the nervous system, and in moderation is generally considered harmless. But it does increase general muscle tension (or *tonus*) and sensitivity to nerve signals of all kinds, including pain. Patients suffering either muscular pain or inflammation are likely to be more comfortable without such extra stimulation. Among common sources of caffeine, coffee is by far the strongest, especially if brewed strong and drunk black. Tea, chocolate, and cola drinks contain far less, but the quantity is not negligible.

There's one other kind of "cane" therapy I give to many patients: advice on harmful postural habits of the kind described in Chapter 3. The most common—and the most harmful—is thrusting the head forward and tilting the chin up. I will discuss these habits in more detail in Chapter 6.

• Medications

I don't hesitate to prescribe painkillers and other medications, especially for patients who are just beginning treatment and are in severe pain. Some practitioners disagree. They argue that pain-relieving medications can mask significant symptoms and that they do nothing to cure the real problems. This is true; patients on medication have to be monitored carefully. But medications can help patients get through the bad times, and I believe that even the temporary relief of pain is a worthwhile objective as long as it forms part of an overall treatment plan.

Some medications are most effective in relieving myofascial pain. Some are more effective against inflammation. Some work on both. They fall into five basic categories:

1. Painkillers, or *analgesics*. These include the familiar Tylenol and aspirin. They help relieve both inflammation and muscular pain. Of all the mild analgesics, I don't know anything better than aspirin. A coated form can be substituted, for those whose stomachs are sensitive to acid.

Only in exceptional cases do I prescribe anything stronger, like codeine or other narcotics, and then only in limited doses for a short period. Codeine is indeed an effective painkiller, especially when used *with* aspirin, but it can be habit-forming and has other undesirable side effects. If you're taking any narcotic or barbiturate, you must avoid alcohol at all costs; the combination of alcohol and drugs can be deadly.

2. *Anti-inflammatory medications*. There are two main groups of these: One group is made up of *corticosteroids*, often simply called steroids. The other is composed of *nonsteroidal* anti-inflammatory medications. The second group is the more commonly used and safer of the two.

One quite useful nonsteroidal anti-inflammatory is good old aspirin. Its double effect—relieving pain and reducing inflammation—is one of the reasons I like to prescribe it. All the nonsteroidal anti-inflammatories, in fact, have some analgesic effects as well.

There's a large family of anti-inflammatories, with new formulations and combinations coming along all the time. They have tongue-twister technical names like ibuprofen, indomethacin, tolmetin, and naproxen. But many of them go by brand names that are more familiar, and certainly easier to pronounce: Motrin for ibuprofen; Indocin for indomethacin; Naprosyn for naproxen. The effects of each vary from patient to patient, and a fair amount of trial and error is often necessary to find one that's effective. For Melissa Sontag's joint inflammation, I found Naprosyn to give the best results.

None of these medications goes to work right away. Their concentration in the blood must be gradually raised to a certain level, a process that usually requires at least three days before any effect at all is apparent. For maximum effectiveness, you have to take the prescribed doses quite religiously for two weeks or more, and not just when you "need" them or "feel like" taking them.

Like aspirin, the medications in this group sometimes upset the stomach. Again, the effect varies from patient to patient. Finding one that isn't irritating has to be part of the trial-and-error process.

Nonsteroidal anti-inflammatories are reasonably safe and easy to use, but they do not work for every patient. In some cases, steroids may be appropriate. TMJ disorders are sometimes treated with the steroid dexamethasone, mixed with an anesthetic like lidocaine and injected next to, or directly into, the inflamed joint. A single shot can provide relief for days, weeks, or even months.

Injected steroids should be used quite sparingly—a good rule of thumb is no more than two injections into the TMJ during a six-month period. Frequent injections can lead to deterioration or even destruction of cartilage and bone tissue in the joint.

3. *Local anesthetics.* These are injected to relieve muscle pain and to break up trigger points. Their names all end in *-caine;* the most commonly used are lidocaine and carbocaine. I describe their use more fully in Chapter 6.

4. *Muscle relaxants.* This is another large and varied group of medications that relax tense muscles and hence are useful in relieving myofascial pain. Examples include methocarbamol (better known by the brand name Robaxin) and orphenadrine citrate (Norgesic). Sometimes they are combined with others for broader usefulness. Norgesic Forte, for instance, contains aspirin and caffeine as well as orphenadrine citrate.

Some of these medications also reduce anxiety and are widely used for that purpose. They include diazepam, more familiarly known as Valium, and chlordiazepoxide, known as Librium. They are especially useful in treating TMJ disorders in which psychological stress is a factor (as it often is). Some patients find that taking one of these medications at bedtime helps them reduce grinding their teeth while they sleep.

Taken over a long period, though, muscle relaxants are habit-forming and can lead to psychological dependency. I don't like to prescribe them for more than a few weeks.

5. *Antidepressants.* A fairly new form of pain-relieving therapy involves medications originally developed to fight emotional depression. One of the better-known antidepressants is amitriptyline—brand name Elavil—but there are many others. They are given to myofascial-pain patients in very low doses—much lower than those used to treat depression. These doses are gradually increased until they take effect on the pain.

• TENS Therapy

There is one other, relatively new tool for relieving joint and muscle pain, especially chronic pain. It is commonly used by dentists, osteopaths, physical therapists, and the like, and is called *transcutaneous electrical nerve stimula-*

tion, or *TENS*. (*Transcutaneous* means "across or through the skin.") TENS passes short pulses of mild electric current through electrodes placed on the skin. These electrical signals "compete" with pain signals and prevent the nerves from transmitting the pain messages to the brain.

Until recently TENS treatment could be given only in a professional office, but now portable units are available for use at home. TENS usually gives only temporary relief—a few hours at most—but it requires no drugs and sometimes works when other methods don't.

• Splints

None of the therapies described so far was originally developed by dentists or for TMJ treatment. All of them are also regularly used by physicians, physical therapists, and others who treat chronic pain. But the next category of treatment, the use of *splints*, very definitely requires dental training, experience, and equipment—one of several reasons the treatment of TMJ disorders is the special province of dentists.

Described bluntly, a splint is a hunk of shaped plastic that slips over the teeth in one jaw. In its most basic form it simply keeps the jaws from closing completely. This might not seem like much of an accomplishment, but in fact it is an important element in the treatment of most TMJ patients. Slightly separating the jaws, for example, tends to rest and relax the fatigued muscles that give rise to myofascial pain. Separation also tends to discourage the habits of clenching and grinding that can lead to disk displacement. And, by keeping the condyles from moving to their deepest positions in the fossae, it can reduce continued irritation of inflamed tissue in the joints.

There are two main types of splints (or *appliances*, as

they're sometimes called). Flat-plane splints separate the jaw, but leave the lower jaw free to close in any position that feels natural and comfortable. Repositioning splints separate the jaws and also direct the lower jaw to a specific position in relation to the upper.

• Flat-Plane Splints

Flat-plane splints are sometimes called *bite plates*, or, if they are to be worn only at night, *night guards*. The very simplest are made of soft rubber or plastic—much like the protective mouthpieces used by athletes. They're certainly easy to make and easy to use, but I don't find them desirable for most patients. They should definitely not be used by patients who habitually clench their teeth: the soft, yielding surface appears to encourage the habit.

Like most other practitioners, I favor splints made of hard acrylic instead. These are made in a wide variety of forms. Some fit over the top teeth, some over the bottom. Some cover all the teeth in the jaw; some cover only a few. Although many a professional meeting has been spent arguing over which kind works best, there's no consensus. Results vary from dentist to dentist and patient to patient.

All such splints are fabricated in much the same way. The one made for Melissa Sontag is typical. During her first visit, I started the process by making molds and casts of her teeth. Over the cast of the lower jaw a dental lab fashioned a horseshoe-shape appliance of acrylic, reinforced with wire. When Ms. Sontag came in again, I trimmed and fitted the splint so that it would slip comfortably over her lower teeth and so that her upper teeth would hit it evenly when she closed her mouth.

The top surface of the appliance was smooth (which is why it's called a *flat-plane* splint). Her upper teeth "skated" freely on it, and her lower jaw was not forced into any particular position when it was closed. That's the biggest difference between this kind of *permissive* splint and the second kind, called a *directive* or *repositioning* splint.

At first, Melissa Sontag wore the splint night and day, except when eating and brushing her teeth. After three weeks, as the inflammation from her injury subsided, she gradually cut back on its use until she was wearing it only at night. Since her problem was only inflammation, she was able to taper off entirely after three months. The usual course of such splint treatment is three to six months. Some patients need longer, and some find they need to return to it from time to time.

Splint therapy is not painful but does take a while for many patients to get used to. The appliance can be fabricated so as to be quite inconspicuous, but initially it may feel rather foreign in the mouth. Some patients report difficulty in speaking clearly, especially if the splint is installed over the upper teeth. Usually, though, the tongue learns to adjust to the new position in three or four days.

Under the combined regimen of cold therapy, anti-inflammatory medication, and a splint, Melissa Sontag's recovery was gradual but steady. Every day she found that she could open her mouth just a little further than the day before. That's about par for the course; no treatment provides instant relief. Also, there's a lot of variation in the time it takes for a particular patient to recover from a specific disorder. Even a patient with a relatively simple problem like this isn't going to feel noticeably better for several days, and complete recovery is likely to take at least a couple of months. For patients with more serious problems, it may take considerably longer for treatment to take hold.

Moreover, a flat-plane splint isn't likely to help two significant groups of patients. The first is patients with displaced articular disks. For them, it is usually not enough to separate the jaws. The mandible may also have to be repositioned in relation to the temporal bones, something a flat-plane appliance can't do.

The second group is patients who suffer muscular pain from severe malocclusion, particularly those who have lost many teeth. As a result their jaws close too far—we say that their bite has lost much of its *vertical dimension.* The separation provided by a flat-plane splint usually doesn't restore enough vertical dimension to put the bite back in balance or relieve the strained chewing muscles.

Nonetheless, for patients like Melissa Sontag I expect successful results and a definite trend of improvement within about two months. And most such patients—about four out of five, or 80 percent—either do recover or show very significant improvement. But that other 20 percent must be re-evaluated. For these patients, as for those with displaced disks or severe malocclusion, it may be necessary to try the second type of splint.

• Repositioning Splints

One morning, without warning, Jane Dudley found that she could hardly open her mouth. After a few hours she was finally able to work her jaw loose from its locked position. A few days later the same thing happened, and meanwhile she became aware of pronounced clicking when she opened and closed her mouth. Soon the joints became increasingly painful as well.

She went to her dentist, who told her she had a TMJ disorder, probably as a result of habitually clenching and grinding her teeth. He gave her a soft rubber splint, which she wore faithfully for several months, but her condition only seemed to get worse. Her jaw continued to lock occasionally, and the pain became more severe despite painkillers and anti-inflammatory drugs.

She asked the advice of a family friend, an orthodontist who happened to be a colleague of mine at Mount Sinai. He referred her to me. When I examined her, it was quite plain that the disks on both sides were badly displaced—squeezed so far forward that they sometimes caused her jaw to lock.

There were two reasons her soft bite plate wasn't working. First, as I've mentioned, a soft appliance often doesn't help someone who habitually clenches the teeth. On the contrary, it seems to encourage the habit and may sometimes make the condition worse. Second, disk displacement is seldom remedied by a permissive, flat-plane splint, which only slightly changes the relationship of the lower jaw to the upper and the position of the condyles in the joints.

What Ms. Dudley needed, and what I gave her, was a repositioning splint, which brought her lower jaw forward when she closed it (Figure 19). This in turn caused the condyles to move forward, to a position where the disks might be "recaptured" and moved back on top of the condyles where they belonged.

A repositioning splint, like a flat-plane splint, may be fitted over either the upper or lower teeth. But the surface facing the other teeth is not smooth; it contains shallow impressions of those teeth. Thus, when the jaws close, the teeth are directed into the impressions on the splint, *repositioning* the mandible into a specific, predetermined position in relation to the upper jaw.

The secret of an effective repositioning splint, of course, is deciding exactly where the jaw should be directed. Several different methods are used to make this determination, and there is no universal agreement about what the ideal placement should be. Most experts agree,

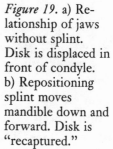

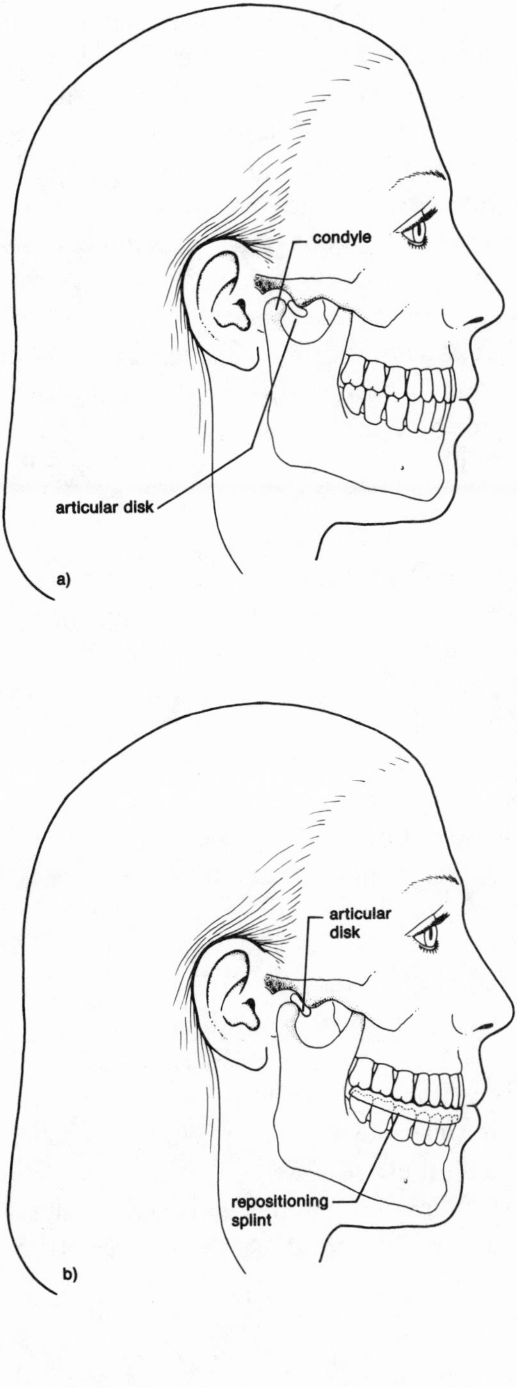

Figure 19. a) Relationship of jaws without splint. Disk is displaced in front of condyle. b) Repositioning splint moves mandible down and forward. Disk is "recaptured."

though, that the condyles should be repositioned somewhat *forward* from their customary location, so they won't "load" the backs of the joints. Virtually all repositioning splints now in use pull the mandible forward in this way.

Like many other practitioners, I don't feel that any particular position is ideal for all patients. Instead, working with the patient, I try to find a position that is likely to recapture the disks. For example, when I was preparing to fit Jane Dudley with a splint, I had her open and close several times, with her lower jaw thrust farther and farther forward, until we found a position that produced no clicking. This in turn indicated that we had arrived at the best location for each condyle in relation to the disk and the temporal fossa.

I then "recorded" this position by having her bite the same way into a sheet of soft wax. A dental lab, using casts of her teeth, fashioned the appliance to match this model.

I sometimes use another method to prepare such a splint. First, a flat-plane splint is made in the usual way, over a cast of the teeth. I then insert that splint in the patient's mouth, with additional soft acrylic applied to its other surface. The patient bites into the soft plastic, in the position already decided on, and holds that position until the plastic sets firm. Thus the patient's own teeth, rather than a separate cast, form the second set of impressions in the splint.

Some practitioners use a somewhat different technique to determine the placement of the mandible. They hook the patient up to a machine called a *myomonitor*. It is similar to the TENS apparatus used to relieve pain, except that the pulses of electricity are repeated more slowly. Applied to the sides of the face, these repeated pulses stimulate the nerves that make the chewing muscles contract, rhythmically closing the jaw. In the process, the electrical impulses override the habitual patterns of the jaw muscles and relax them.

After about forty-five minutes of such pulsing, the lower jaw is so relaxed that it hangs open slackly. The dentist then inserts a flat-plane splint, with additional soft acrylic on the second surface. Further electrical stimulation is applied, again causing the jaw to close in a repeated, rhythmical pattern. The position of the facing teeth is thus impressed into the soft plastic. The proponents of this method maintain that the resulting splint provides the best possible relationship of the condyles with the disks and temporal bones.

When I fitted Jane Dudley for her splint, I told her what I tell all patients beginning this kind of therapy. She would be wearing the splint from three to six months. There was about an 80 percent chance that her symptoms would significantly diminish. But the splint wouldn't really cure her problems, and once she stopped wearing it and her bite returned to its usual position, the symptoms might return.

For more permanent relief, I went on, she might have to undertake *phase-two* treatment to establish her bite in the new position. One possibility would be restorative dentistry. This might be nothing more than grinding the surfaces of certain teeth so they would meet properly in the new biting position. Or it might mean building up certain teeth with crowns, or installing bridgework to replace missing teeth.

The second alternative would be orthodontics—using braces and other devices to move her teeth into the proper position. Unlike splint therapy, both these phase-two treatments would be essentially irreversible.

Finally I cautioned her that the splint therapy just might not work. It might not succeed in recapturing the disks or in relieving her symptoms. In that unlikely event, she might have to consider another alternative—surgery on one or both joints or on the jaw.

However, the repositioning splint worked remarkably well in Ms. Dudley's case. In six months she was almost completely free of pain and could open her mouth normally. I concluded that the disk had indeed been recaptured and was no longer displaced. But it was also evident that the cure wouldn't be permanent unless something was done about her malocclusion. Along with her clenching and grinding habit, this seemed a basic cause of her disorder. The teeth didn't meet properly, throwing her bite off balance. Sooner or later the symptoms were likely to return. So she then went back to the orthodontist.

I describe orthodontics and other forms of phase-two treatment in Chapter 8. But in Chapters 6 and 7 I want to discuss two other types of therapy that often form part of phase-one treatment: physical therapy, and treatment for psychological stress.

SIX

Team Effort

THE ROLE OF PHYSICAL THERAPY

Margaret Finch, who came to me just after finishing her first year of college, had for several years suffered periodically from a variety of aches and pains in her head and neck. Her temples would ache, or she would feel pressure behind her eyes, accompanied by blurred vision. Her tongue would feel thick and raw. The muscles of her neck, especially near the back of her head, would become stiff and sore, and her hands would become numb. The preceding winter she had begun to have severe earaches. An ear-nose-throat specialist found no sign of disease and referred her to me for examination.

To me it was plain that Margaret's wide-ranging symptoms were mainly related to myofascial pain from a TMJ disorder. I suspected that the original cause was an uneven bite. I started her on phase-one treatment, prescribing a mild relaxant medication and making a flat-plane splint that would also tend to relax the chewing muscles. But I felt that her symptoms called for other treatment as well.

"The splint I'm making for you should start relieving some of your symptoms over the next few days," I told her. "The headaches and earaches should certainly taper off. Probably that thick, tingly feel in your tongue as well. But the pain and stiffness you get in your neck muscles and the numbness in your hands—well, they're related to your TMJ problem, but they could use some attention on their own. For instance, are you aware that you have a habit of pushing your head forward and your chin out?"

"I hadn't noticed," Margaret said. "But now that you mention it, I guess I do. Is that a problem?

"It can be, by itself," I replied. "Or it can make other problems worse. For instance, it might be what's causing the numbness in your hands. I'd like to send you to a colleague of mine, a physical therapist. I think he could give you some relief from your symptoms. But just as important, I think, he could help you get rid of what we call trigger points, which carry pain to different muscles. And he could help you with your posture, and give you a program of exercise that would keep the pain from coming back. Are you willing to give it a try?"

"Sure," she said.

TMJ disorders, as I've already stressed, aren't like the measles, which can be treated by a single physician, or like an abscessed tooth, which can be treated by a single dentist. Instead, their treatment often requires a team effort by practitioners in several different fields. The dentist serves as coordinator of treatment as a whole but must often rely on colleagues with special knowledge and experience different from his own.

Some of these colleagues provide advanced, phase-two treatment, such as oral surgery and orthodontics, which I'll discuss later. But even during primary, phase-one treatment, the dentist often collaborates with other professionals in at least two fields. One is physical therapy, which I prescribed for Margaret Finch. The other is treatment of psychological conditions, which often accompany

TMJ disorders or contribute to them. I'll discuss that in Chapter 7.

• What Is Physical Therapy?

Physical therapy plays an important role in treating several kinds of TMJ disorders, but it is especially useful with myofascial pain. It has two main goals: the relief of pain and the restoration of function, particularly the function of movement. In addition, it often helps patients develop weak or underused muscles and improve their posture and other physical habits.

Some dentists include physical-therapy procedures in their own treatment program—I do so myself. But when the therapy is likely to be extensive, or when it involves parts of the body (like Ms. Finch's neck and back muscles) relatively far from the TMJ itself, many dentists prefer to send the patient to a separate therapist.

Ordinarily a physical therapist is not what is called a *primary care provider*. Instead, patients must be *referred* to a therapist by a physician or dentist. Nonetheless, such a therapist is a licensed health professional and trained both to evaluate and to treat many kinds of bone and muscle ailments.

Consequently, the first time a patient goes for physical therapy, the therapist very likely will (like a physician or dentist) take a complete medical history, review other medical records such as X-rays, perform a thorough physical examination, and come up with a plan of treatment suited to that individual patient and his or her specific problems.

The therapist has a wide repertory of techniques to choose from. Usually treatment concentrates first on reducing pain and inflammation, and after that on restoring mobility. Sometimes, though, the two goals are pursued at the same time.

• Heat and Cold

When Margaret Finch went to the physical therapist, one of the first treatments he gave her was the application of heat to the sore muscles of her head, neck, and back. Heat and cold are of course among the oldest remedies for pain and still rank among the most effective. Anyone who has dissolved a muscle cramp under a warm shower can testify to that, as can anyone who has put a hammer-mashed thumb into a bowl of ice.

Heat and cold therapies work in rather different ways. Cold tends to slow down the activities of cells. It makes inflamed cells, such as those in the synovial lining of the TMJ, less hyperactive, and it helps relax muscle spasms. Cold also serves as an anesthetic, dulling pain sensations in joint and muscle cells.

Heat tends to work more indirectly. Pain, especially muscle pain, is often caused by a relative shortage of oxygen in the tissues, which allows the buildup of metabolic waste products like lactic acid. This *oxygen debt* is usually produced by fatigue. Heat applied to the tissues tends to dilate the blood vessels passing through them. This increases the blood flow and hence carries more oxygen to the tissues. The oxygen debt is reduced, the lactic acid is dispersed and the pain diminishes.

Cold therapy tends to be used particularly to relieve inflammation. In the preceding chapter I described how I used it to alleviate Melissa Sontag's trauma-produced capsulitis and retrodiscitis. Heat, on the other hand, tends to be used more for muscle pain like Margaret Finch's. But there is no fixed rule for when to use heat and when to use cold—some patients simply respond better to one or the other, regardless of the type of pain. Furthermore, heat and cold can be used together. Some therapists use a cold application to diminish pain sensations, then follow with heat to bring more oxygen to the tissues.

Heat therapy can take several different forms. The simplest is the old-fashioned moist compress, such as a towel soaked in hot water. A hot-water bottle applied over the compress makes it stay warm longer. Many professionals use a device called a Hydrocolator (sounds like "percolator"), a wrapper made of soft fabric, with a pocket for a bag of heat-retaining fluid. The wrapper can be placed around the shoulders, neck, or head, and is held in place with Velcro fasteners.

Two sophisticated mechanical techniques are used to penetrate painful areas deep within the tissues. One is *ultrasound*, which uses a machine to generate sound waves at frequencies too high to be heard by the human ear. Directed through living tissue, ultrasound stimulates the cells and causes them to vibrate and give off heat.

The second technique, called *electrogalvanic stimulation* (*EGS*), works on the cells by running a mild electric current through them. This current doesn't heat the tissues but does produce one of the effects of heat therapy: It tends to contract muscle fibers and to encourage the flow of oxygen-rich blood through them. Until fairly recently ultrasound and EGS machines were available only in professional facilities, but now portable models have been developed that patients can use at home.

The simplest and most common cold therapy is the application of ice. Perhaps the easiest method is to seal the ice in a plastic bag that is then wrapped in a dry towel. You can also use a ready-made cold pack, which retains some flexibility even if chilled to a temperature below that of ice. Also available are so-called *snap-packs*, which don't even have to be chilled. Striking them on a hard surface sets off a chemical reaction that makes them lose heat quickly.

One caution about ice or other cold therapy: don't use it for very long at a time. The usual rule is no more than twenty minutes in any hour, and you should stop immediately if the skin looks unnaturally pale.

• TENS and Massage

The physical therapist uses a number of other techniques to relieve pain. One is transcutaneous electrical nerve stimulation (TENS). As noted in Chapter 5, the TENS machine conducts an electric current through painful tissue such as sore muscles. This current has a different frequency from that of EGS, and instead of stimulating the tissue the electrical impulses act upon the nerves and override pain signals to the central nervous system. Thus, at least temporarily, the patient doesn't "feel" the pain.

TENS electrodes are also sometimes attached to the sides of the head, and current is run through the scalp and muscle tissues encasing the skull. The process is called *transcranial* TENS, and it is thought to encourage the release of certain chemicals that naturally diminish pain sensations.

Incidentally, even the temporary relief of pain can have long-range benefits. It can help break what therapists call the *pain cycle*. Spasms in the muscles cause compression of the nerve tissues, resulting in muscular pain. But then the pain provokes *further* spasms, which produce more pain, and so the cycle continues. Breaking the cycle at any point can lead to a general reduction of symptoms.

Another form of pain-relieving therapy is of very great

antiquity: massage. Massage is particularly effective in treating muscular pain. Like EGS, it encourages the flow of blood through the tissues and reduces their oxygen debt. Massage also helps cramped, spastic muscles regain their mobility.

To relieve Margaret Finch's sore head, neck, and back muscles, the therapist followed heat applications with massage, both longitudinally (along the muscle fibers) and transversely (across them). To increase mobility, he also used *contract-and-stretch* massage. He first manipulated a specific set of muscles to make them contract. Next he allowed them to relax briefly, then stretched them out to their fullest length.

He also gave her a relatively new form of tissue manipulation called *myofascial release*. This technique is based on the theory that myofascial pain results not only from spasms in the muscle fibers but also from constrictions in the *fascia*, the connective tissue wrapped around the muscles and woven into them. Fascia is composed of stringy fibers of the protein *collagen*, which makes up more than half the solid content of the musculoskeletal system.

Those who practice myofascial release maintain that a constriction in fascia can be felt under the skin by an experienced therapist. The therapist gently but firmly presses the area overlying such a constriction for anywhere from ninety seconds to several minutes. Eventually the constriction "releases," and regular massage may be used to relax and disperse it further.

For example, to relieve soreness in the masseter muscles of the jaw, of the kind that Margaret Finch suffered from, the therapist first holds the jaw firmly closed, putting the masseters into their most contracted form without any voluntary tensing by the patient. Then he or she applies very gentle pressure in the opposite direction—

down the masseters—until the restriction in the fascia releases. The mouth spontaneously opens, stretching the muscles and relaxing them.

• Trigger-Point Therapy

Trigger points are muscle areas—usually small, but sometimes fairly extensive—that form in persistently constricted tissue and tend to trigger pain sensations elsewhere in the body. Physical therapists are trained to locate these areas and break them up. It is one of the most important aspects of their work.

Specific trigger points in one muscle tend to refer pain to specific areas in others. From the nature of Margaret Finch's pains, the physical therapist had a pretty good idea where to look for the trigger points that caused them. For example, her symptoms included earaches, and pain in the ear is often referred from one or more trigger points deep in the masseter muscle of the jaw. She also suffered from headaches in her temples and at the base of her skull. These can be referred from trigger points in the coat-hanger-shaped trapezius muscle at the top of the back. Such trigger points commonly result from the strain of a forward-head posture like hers.

An experienced therapist can often locate the hardened knots of trigger points simply by touch. Some also use a special version of TENS called a *neuroprobe*. In this mode, the electrode is used as a sensor rather than a stimulator. As the electrode is passed over the skin, the machine registers the amount of resistance to the current created by the skin and underlying muscles. Wherever a sharp drop in resistance occurs, a constricted trigger point is likely to be lurking in the muscle.

Once a trigger point is located with the probe, the machine can be switched to the customary TENS mode, conducting a stimulating current through the electrode. "Zapping" the nearby nerve ends can give quick, if temporary, relief from the pain the trigger point produces, and can help break the "pain cycle" I described earlier.

The most common of all physical therapies for trigger points is called *stretch and spray*, but might more accurately be labeled "spray and stretch," since the spray comes first. The spray is a highly volatile liquid—often ethyl chloride. When it hits the skin, it evaporates quickly, chilling and partly numbing the skin. The patient is instructed to relax the muscle as much as possible, and the therapist then slowly stretches it to its fullest extension. During the process, trigger points in the muscle are broken up and dispersed. Heat treatment is often used as a follow-up to restore and increase circulation. Relief from pain can be dramatic and often long-lasting.

I should also mention one form of trigger-point treatment that is *not* performed by physical therapists, since it requires injections, which only dentists and physicians are licensed to dispense. This therapy is especially useful in locating and treating trigger points in relatively deep and inaccessible tissues such as the pterygoid muscles inside the jaw.

The target muscle is injected with a local anesthetic, such as lidocaine. The injection will certainly make that muscle less tender, but if it relieves referred pain elsewhere as well, you can be fairly sure that the muscle contains one or more trigger points. The anesthetic injection, furthermore, sometimes appears to break up these trigger points, giving long-term relief.

For an identifiable trigger point close to the skin, a "blank" injection is sometimes used instead. That is, a dry needle is inserted directly into the constricted knot of muscle. Sometimes this counterirritation is all that's needed to break it up.

• Exercise and Other Aids to Mobility

Many of the techniques used by the physical therapist are designed not only to relieve muscular pain but also to restore function, or *mobility*. Mobility has two aspects. One is the capacity for smooth, unobstructed movement, commonly described as *suppleness*. The other is the capacity of the muscles to keep the body stable and to perform work efficiently—the balanced strength called *muscle tone*.

If muscles are to be mobile they must be exercised. Just about every program of physical therapy includes a prescribed regimen of exercises, concentrating on the parts of the body most affected. In Margaret Finch's case, these were the head and throat muscles directly involved with her TMJs and also the other muscles of her neck and upper back.

Some exercises are designed to stretch the muscles for greater suppleness; others are meant to strengthen them for better muscle tone. Exercises are useful not only in relieving specific disorders, but also in generally maintaining the muscles in smooth, efficient working order. In case you'd like to try out a few exercises for suppleness of the head and neck muscles, I've included a short series on the next page.

As already indicated, measures to improve mobility, especially exercises, must often come after those designed to relieve pain. And exercises to stretch the muscles must often precede those that build strength. Finally, no exercise should be so prolonged, or so intense, that it *produces* pain. The general rule is "If it hurts, don't do it."

EXERCISES FOR THE HEAD AND NECK MUSCLES TO INCREASE SUPPLENESS

Do all of the following either standing or sitting erect.

1. With your head held erect, tuck in your chin as much as possible, as if you were trying to push it toward the back of your neck. Hold the tucked position for two or three seconds, then relax your head to its original position. Repeat five times. (This exercise is useful in overcoming the postural fault of thrusting the head forward.)
2. Fold your arms, with your elbows held slightly away from your body. Rotate your head to the left, and at the same time rotate your arms to the right. Hold that position for two seconds, then rotate your head to the right and your arms to the left. Again, hold the position for two seconds. Return your arms and head to the center position, and relax. Repeat five times.
3. Rotate your head 45 degrees toward your left shoulder. Lower your head until you feel a stretch in the muscles of the back of your neck, particularly on the right side. Hold that position for five seconds. Then rotate your head to the right side and repeat the process. Return your head to an erect central position, and relax. Repeat the exercise five times.
4. In a slow, even rhythm, gently roll your head and upper neck above the shoulders. Make the roll oval rather than circular—extending farther from side to side than front to back—and don't tip your head back very far. Repeat eight times in each direction.

• Posture Correction

For many physical therapists, a large proportion of treatment time is devoted to correcting posture problems. As one therapist points out, "Poor posture is a pre-existing irritant" to muscular pain disorders. "As long as it is not corrected, the patient will never really get better."

Margaret Finch suffered from the most common, and the most harmful, of postural faults—the head thrust forward and the chin tilted up. I described it earlier as "bird-watcher's posture," but it is very common among students and all sorts of clerical workers who must give close visual attention to work in front of them. It also afflicts those who watch television while lying down and those who habitually slump when sitting.

The most common and generally most effective form of posture re-education is simply increasing awareness. Once the patient is aware of the problem, it is usually not difficult to correct it. At first the patient will only correct the unhealthy habit when thinking about it, but gradually this conscious correction will become translated into a new, healthy habit.

Posture training covers four main categories: standing posture, sitting posture, lying posture, and habitual positions and activities that strain certain muscles.

- *Standing posture.* There is more to good posture than simply "standing up straight." Yes, it is desirable to keep the head erect and the shoulders back—within limits. An exaggerated military posture, chest thrust forward and chin held rigidly in, is almost as harmful as a forward slump. The chest and shoulders should be as relaxed as possible, and the head should be balanced without strain at the top of the neck.

The noted physician Janet Travell recommends a simple but effective way to assure good standing posture, using the weight distribution of the body. Instead of standing with your weight concentrated over your heels, rock forward slightly so your weight is mainly on the balls of your feet. As the weight of your lower body shifts forward, your head and shoulders will naturally settle back to serve as a balancing counterweight. In fact, if you try to thrust your head forward in this position, you'll slowly but surely fall on your face.

• *Sitting posture.* Warning: chairs may be dangerous to your health. Unless they are specially designed, they probably won't support the middle and lower parts of the back but will encourage slumping instead. One remedy is to insert a small pillow or cushion between your back and the chair, just above the waistline, in order to provide the missing support. It also helps not to sit cross-legged or in one position for a long time without a break.

Driving presents additional problems. If the seat is pushed too far back or is too low in relationship to the dashboard, you're likely to thrust your head forward, craning to see the road. If the seat is tilted too far from vertical, you may be inclined to hunch your body forward. If the seat is adjustable, check and correct its position every time you drive. If it's not, extra cushions under or behind you can sometimes provide the needed change.

• *Lying posture.* One big no-no here: lying on your stomach, with your head twisted to one side. This is hard on virtually every muscle and joint, from back to head. Almost as bad is lying on your back, with your head propped up at a sharp angle for reading or watching television.

The healthiest and most restful lying position is on the side, with a pillow thick enough to support the head and neck horizontally and the arms and legs loosely flexed. There are special orthopedic pillows available, such as the cylindrical Jackson neck roll and others, that provide this kind of support. But many therapists recommend simply a good, plump down pillow for the job.

• *Things to avoid.* There are several specific positions

and activities that fatigue muscles and either cause or contribute to pain:

—Cradling the telephone between shoulder and chin.

—Propping the chin on one or both hands for extended periods.

—Reaching high over the head for a burden. Also painting, hammering, or doing other work on high walls or ceilings.

—Carrying a heavy shoulder bag on the same shoulder for an extended period.

—Wearing high-heeled boots or shoes.

• Physical Therapy after Surgery

Physical therapy is a crucial element of one other aspect of medical care: recovery from surgery. Its most important function is keeping fibrotic scar tissue from interfering with joint and muscle mobility. (I will refer to this again in Chapter 9.)

Margaret Finch's TMJ disorder responded quickly and readily to the program that combined splint therapy with physical therapy. She began to experience relief within a week, and after seven weeks was able to discontinue the physical therapy. She continued to wear the splint at night for an additional three months—more as a precaution than as a necessity. She still has a malocclusion that may require attention later on. But right now, a year later, she is free of pain and able to lead a normal life.

SEVEN

COPING WITH PSYCHOLOGICAL STRESS

At the very beginning of this book, I told part of the story of Joy Forrester, who came to me after months of vainly seeking treatment for severe headaches. I was able to verify the suspicion of her allergist that she was suffering from a TMJ disorder. She had both joint inflammation and muscle pain as a result of a displaced disk in the right TMJ. I put her on a course of phase-one treatment, including a repositioning splint, and her symptoms began to subside in a little over a week.

But it was plain to me that, although I was relieving the symptoms, I wasn't getting at the sources of her troubles. One of these sources was malocclusion. Her lower jaw was relatively narrow, and the lower teeth met the upper ones too far back. The repositioning splint moved the jaw forward, taking some of the load off the joint and recapturing the disk. But I knew that she would eventually need orthodontics—phase-two treatment—to correct the condition permanently.

A more immediate problem was the obvious tension in her chewing muscles. She admitted that she habitually clenched her teeth, and there was visible evidence of the overdeveloped masseter muscles that sometimes result from this habit (we call it the "chipmunk face" syndrome).

Clenching not only produces muscle fatigue and pain directly, it also leads to disk displacement in one or both of the joints. As I said earlier, the mechanics of this process are still not completely understood, but when the jaw clenches shut, forces from the muscles apparently shift the disk forward until it is eventually displaced in front of the condyle. Joy Forrester had already reached the stage where the disk in the right TMJ was partially displaced, causing noticeable clicking when she opened and closed her mouth.

The clenching habit often represents a response to psychological stress, and Ms. Forrester exhibited fairly high levels of anxiety and nervous tension. These resulted in part from her demanding job in a fast-paced corporation and in part from the physical pain she had been suffering. But they also seemed to originate from her basic personal makeup; indeed, she described herself as "rather high-strung." I believed that, like many TMJ patients, she would benefit from treatment to help her cope more effectively with stress. I therefore referred her to a clinical psychologist, one who concentrates upon behavioral therapy in treating stress-related disorders.

• The "Fight or Flight" Response

To understand how behavioral therapy works, you may find helpful a commonly used explanation for the way human beings respond to stress. The human nervous system is several million years old, and built into it is a mechanism for protection from imminent danger through the immediate output of physical energy. Psychologists call this the "fight or flight" response: the body automatically responds to the perception of danger with preparations either to defend itself or to run away.

Specifically, the threat of danger triggers production of the hormone adrenalin, which speeds up the heartbeat and rate of breathing and increases muscle tension. This automatic mechanism was an effective response to immediate physical peril, like an attack by a saber-toothed tiger. It built up energy in the body, which was then dissipated by fighting or escaping.

But today human beings live in a world in which few problems can be solved in those ways. The mechanism still works—we still respond to stress with a buildup of physical energy, regardless of the cause and nature of that stress. But usually the stresses of modern life don't come from physical perils and cannot be dissipated by fight or flight. "When I worry about paying the rent," says one psychologist, "my body responds as if my life is in physical danger. But I can't run away from my problems or throw a spear at them."

As a result, the energy created in response to stress tends to accumulate in the body. Eventually it seeks an outlet. It often finds some constitutional "weak link," which will vary from one individual to another. Thus one person may respond to stress with a "nervous" headache, another with "nervous" indigestion. And some will respond with certain behavior habits—like clenching or grinding the teeth.

Individuals respond to stress in different ways and to different degrees. Those who suffer from stress-related disorders tend to have relatively low tolerance to its pressures. There's no single "personality profile" for such patients, but many of them do seem to share certain traits. They are sensitive and anxious, with high personal standards and a strong sense of responsibility. They tend to mask their powerful emotions under a calm surface. They are often the individuals others turn to for leadership and help because they seem so composed and self-assured. Underneath, they are anything but, and stress exacts a heavy toll on them.

Also, severely stressful situations or events can often serve as "the straw that broke the camel's back"—triggering disorders in just about anyone. Every half year an unusual number of college students come to me for treatment. Why the sudden increase? It's exam time. Also, several of my patients have started suffering symptoms during a divorce or after the death of someone dear to them.

In Joy Forrester's case, the triggering situation may have been a job change, which took place a couple of months before her physical problems erupted. Her new position was more challenging but also much more pressured, with a faster pace and a very demanding boss. She was beginning to doubt that the challenge was worth the pressure, especially when she became aware that the pain in her head and jaw was probably related to her stress.

The wide variety of treatment offered for stress-related disorders ranges from psychotherapy to behavior modification. Simple behavioral therapy often proves effective to treat the heightened muscle tension and the clenching and grinding habits of TMJ patients, but many other approaches are also used successfully.

• Relaxation Exercises

A major goal of behavioral treatment is teaching the body to relax, or rather teaching it new *habits* of relaxation, which will reduce the strength of the stress response and help the body react to it in less harmful ways. Two basic strategies are used to induce relaxation—one direct, the other indirect.

The direct strategy is a program of relaxation "exercises" for patients to do at home. The first is a simple but surprisingly effective breathing exercise. It serves as an "instant tranquilizer" that can be practiced just about anywhere, any time:

- Inhale slowly and deeply, counting up to five at one-second intervals. Between each count, think of a single word, such as *calm*, or *peace*, to help free your mind of distracting or stressful thoughts.
- Hold your breath for one second, then exhale slowly, counting backward from five to one, and silently repeat your chosen word. At the same time, let your chest and stomach muscles relax, and drop your shoulders.
- Repeat this cycle three times.

The breathing exercise becomes a prelude for a longer series of exercises called *progressive relaxation*. This is a system first developed by psychologist Edmund Jacobson in 1938 and later adapted by many other therapists. Some professionals "walk through" the exercises with each patient, recording them on tape as they do so. The tape is then used as a guide, enabling the patient to go through the program without thinking about what should come next or how long should be spent on each step.

These exercises are quite simple: The patient simply tenses and then relaxes groups of related muscles in progression, over the whole body. There is no set order, but the series often starts at the hands (making a fist), proceeds to the feet (curling the toes), and ends at the head (wrinkling the forehead). Tensing the muscles before relaxing them results in a greater degree of relaxation than just trying to relax them.

While relaxing each group of muscles, the patient is advised to visualize one or more of the following processes:

- Letting *gravity* take control so that the affected area "hangs loose"
- *Smoothing* the area to get rid of any kinks or wrinkles
- *Letting go* the muscles so they don't "hold on"

A typical series of progressive relaxation exercises is reproduced at the end of this chapter. They are meant to be performed daily, in uninterrupted sessions lasting fifteen to thirty minutes.

Some therapists believe that these exercises are most effective when carried out under their direct supervision, in person or on tape. Other practitioners believe that simpler methods will suffice. The patient can work directly from printed instructions or use the instructions to record a cassette at home. Commercially produced cassettes are also available. Finally, for anyone who prefers personal instruction, these exercises are included in many short courses in relaxation and meditation offered by schools, colleges, health clubs, and the like.

• Guided Imagery

The direct strategy of exercise is often paralleled by an indirect strategy called *guided imagery,* designed to train the mind as progressive relaxation is designed to train the body.

Guided imagery induces relaxation by calling up to "the mind's eye" a series of soothing and pleasant sensory images. Either the therapist or the patient develops a mental image of a pleasant, tranquil experience to which the patient's attention is consciously guided. At first it is used just for training, to reduce the level of emotional tension. But, like the breathing exercise or progressive relaxation, it eventually becomes habitual and can be used to provide relief in stressful life situations.

The choice of imagery varies greatly from individual to individual; what relaxes one person might cause another to tense up. Many people find it enjoyable and relaxing to go to the beach, so this is probably the most common choice. But for those who associate the beach with thoughts of sharks, some other location would be better. In any event, the therapist or the patient creates a scenario full of concrete, sensory details, along these lines:

> The scene is a quiet beach on a sunny summer day. The weather is warm, but not hot, because of a gentle, cooling sea breeze. The sand feels warm and soothing between the toes. Overhead, a few fleecy clouds drift through a brilliant blue sky. In the distance, near the horizon, two small sailboats tack back and forth, so far away they barely seem to be moving at all. The waves break on the shore in a slow, regular rhythm. They send shallow flows of foamy water up the sloping sand and carry the scent of salt and seaweed. As the surf ebbs and flows, small sea birds dart back and forth in the shallows. . . .

Such a description can be extended to last several minutes. Like the instructions for relaxation exercises, it can be recorded on a cassette, to be used at home until it is memorized and recalled at will. A session of guided imagery can take place either before or after a series of relaxation exercises. Each reinforces the other.

• Biofeedback

In order to reinforce the relaxation training and heighten the patient's self-awareness, therapists also make use of a special mechanical technique called *biofeedback*.

A biofeedback machine is essentially an electronic amplifier of weak electrical signals. Its input is an electrode, attached to some part of the body and used to record electrically any of several physical changes related to levels of stress. One type, for example, is attached to a finger and measures slight changes in temperature; relative coldness indicates stress while relative warmth indicates relaxation. Another type, which measures the capacity of the skin to conduct electricity, is called *galvanic skin response* (*GSR*). This capacity is affected by perspiration, so the electrode is attached to the palm of the hand. The sweatier the palm, the more stress.

For the treatment of stress-related muscle disorders, many therapists prefer the method that directly measures variations in muscle activity. This method is called *electromyography* (*EMG*). The input electrode is attached to the skin over a particular muscle or muscle group. One of the most commonly used is the frontalis muscle of the forehead. Every time the muscle contracts, even slightly, it generates low-level electrical impulses. The impulses are picked up by the electrode and transmitted to the machine, which amplifies them.

The strengthened signals are then transformed into visible or audible output (or both). Visible output may take the form of flashing lights or a moving dial; audible output may take the form of a tone of varying frequencies or beeps repeated at varying intervals. The stronger and more sustained the muscle contractions, the stronger the impulses picked up by the input electrode and the stronger the output signals. Thus the machine "feeds back" information about the user's level of muscle activity.

The biofeedback machine does more than reflect the amount of activity in the frontalis muscle. The nerves and muscles of the body form a complex, interwoven system. Measuring the activity of certain specific muscles, like the frontalis, can give a revealing picture of the tension level in the system as a whole.

Actually, the biofeedback machine doesn't *do* anything except provide information. But during the last fifteen years or so that it has been in use, it has demonstrated the capacity to reinforce relaxation training to a very remarkable degree, even though the patient may not be consciously aware of its effect.

It also measures the patient's progress, from beginning to end of treatment. When Joy Forrester first used the machine, for instance, her muscles were extremely tense. As she describes it, "The needle just about went off the gauge." After several months of therapy she found herself able to keep her level of response to a very low level—and without thinking very much about it.

Many therapists introduce their patients to the machine at the very first session. At one time, patients used to be quite leery of this process. But possibly as a result of experience with portable cassette players and video games, most now actually enjoy being attached to the machine and interacting with it.

Ordinarily no specific exercises are used with biofeedback. Instead, the therapist instructs the patient simply to concentrate attention on one group of muscles at a time, and to *think* of them as relaxed but not to *try* to relax them.

The patient customarily starts with three main muscle groups at the top of the body—the muscles of the forehead, the jaw, and the shoulders—and then moves on to the rest. As in progressive relaxation, the patient should imagine the muscles yielding to gravity, going limp, smoothing out, or letting go. And while going through this mental process, the patient should simply observe the effect on the machine, rather than consciously try to reduce its output.

The first session, in particular, is devoted to getting acquainted with the machine. Once patients find out what processes seem best able to reduce muscle activity they become aware of how they think and feel at that time. The aim is to give them the ability to accomplish the same kind of relaxation when they are not on the machine.

Eventually, with daily practice of tape-programmed exercises and the reinforcement of biofeedback, the ability to relax the muscles and nervous system becomes a habit. The body has learned to respond to stress in a less hyperactive way. One therapist compares the process to learning a game like tennis. You first get instructions on how to execute the strokes, but you finally learn to play without consciously thinking about them.

Although many psychologists and other mental-health therapists provide behavioral therapy in their courses of treatment, not all of them include biofeedback. Those trained in this technique are certified by the Biofeedback Society of America. The Association for the Advancement of Behavioral Therapy can also provide references. These organizations' addresses appear in the Appendix.

The usual course of relaxation and biofeedback therapy lasts about six months, starting with weekly sessions and then tapering off. Most patients experience at least some relief from nervous tension in four to six weeks. The treatment is effective for a large majority of those who undertake it wholeheartedly. The most common reason for lack of success is the patient's unwillingness to continue to the end or to do the exercises regularly.

That's what happened to Joy Forrester, at least at first. She started in with relaxation exercises and biofeedback but dropped out of the program because splint therapy seemed to be taking care of her symptoms, and she thought other treatment was unnecessary. But after about six months the headaches and other pains she had suffered began to return. The splint didn't give complete relief. So she returned for continued behavioral therapy.

This time she stuck to it for several months. Biofeedback monitoring then showed that her level of nervous tension, which originally had almost "driven the needle off the gauge," was down by more than half. She also found the relaxation exercises very helpful, not only in reducing her overall level of tension but in helping her cope with particularly stressful situations as well. And her symptoms subsided so that she could go on with the phase-two treatment she needed in order to achieve permanent relief from her TMJ disorder.

It must be acknowledged that the kind of relaxation therapy I have been describing here largely treats *symptoms* rather than *causes*. In many cases, that's quite enough. Sometimes, though, the symptoms have their roots in neuroses and other deep-seated personality disorders, which must be addressed if recovery is to be achieved. It lies beyond the scope of this book to explore such problems in detail. In my own practice, whenever I sense that they are present and that they are impeding progress in treatment, I suggest that the patient consider other psychological treatment, such as more intensive behavioral therapy or psychotherapy, to attack these root causes.

PROGRESSIVE RELAXATION EXERCISES

You can perform these exercises either lying down or sitting back in an easy chair. You should do them in a quiet environment with your eyes closed and your clothes loosened if necessary.

About thirty seconds should be devoted to each exercise: ten seconds for tensing each group of muscles, twenty seconds for relaxing. Repeat each exercise twice.

PROGRESSIVE RELAXATION EXERCISES (cont.)

1. Make a tight fist with your left hand. Hold this tense position. Feel the cramped tightness in your palm and fingers.

Now relax your hand. Let your fingers go limp. Let the tension drain away through your fingertips. Feel the warm, comfortable sensation of relaxing.

(Repeat this exercise, then follow the same procedure with the right hand.)

2. Curl the toes of your left foot toward the bottom of your foot. Hold this tense position. Feel the cramped tightness in the sole of your foot and your ankle.

Now relax your foot. Let your toes relax. Let the tension drain from your toes. Feel the warm, comfortable sensation of relaxing.

(Repeat this exercise, then follow the same procedure with the right foot.)

3. Pull the toes of your left foot toward your face. Hold this tense position. Feel the cramped tightness in your calf and knee.

Now relax the foot. Let the tension drain from your leg. Feel the warm, comfortable sensation of relaxing.

(Repeat this exercise, then follow the same procedure with the right leg.)

4. Tense the muscles in your left thigh by pressing your left leg hard against your right leg. Hold this tense position. Feel the cramped tightness in your leg.

PROGRESSIVE RELAXATION EXERCISES (cont.)

Now relax your thigh muscles. Let the tension drain from your leg. Feel the warm, comfortable sensation of relaxing.

(Repeat this exercise, then follow the same procedure with the right thigh.)

5. Imagine that you are sitting on a bed of nails and tighten the muscles of your buttocks by pulling them toward each other. Hold this tense position. Feel the cramped tightness in your buttocks and lower back.

Now imagine that the nails have been removed and relax your buttock muscles. Let the tension drain from your lower back. Feel the warm, comfortable sensation of relaxing.

(Repeat this exercise.)

6. Tighten the muscles of your stomach as if you were trying to protect yourself from being punched. Hold this tense position. Feel the cramped tightness in your abdomen.

Now relax your stomach muscles. Let the tension drain from your abdomen. Feel the warm, comfortable sensation of relaxing.

(Repeat this exercise.)

7. Pull your shoulder blades toward each other. Hold this tense position. Feel the cramped tightness in your back and chest.

PROGRESSIVE RELAXATION EXERCISES (cont.)

Now relax your shoulder blades. Let the tension drain from your back and chest. Feel the warm, comfortable sensation of relaxing.

(Repeat this exercise.)

8. Hunch your shoulders toward your ears. Hold this tense position. Feel the cramped tightness in your shoulders.

Now relax your shoulders. Let them drop. Feel the tension drain away. Feel the warm, comfortable sensation of relaxing.

(Repeat this exercise.)

9. Press the upper part of your left arm hard against your side. Hold this tense position. Feel the cramped tightness in your arm.

Now relax the arm muscles. Let the tension drain away. Feel the warm, comfortable sensation of relaxing.

(Repeat this exercise with the left arm, then follow the same procedure with the right arm.)

10. Push the back of your head hard against the floor or chair to tighten your neck muscles. Hold this tense position. Feel the cramped tightness in your neck.

Now relax your head. Feel the tension drain from your neck. Feel the warm, comfortable sensation of relaxing.

(Repeat this exercise.)

11. Clench your teeth together, push your tongue against

PROGRESSIVE RELAXATION EXERCISES (cont.)

the roof of your mouth, and smile to expose as many teeth as you can. Hold this tense position. Feel the cramped tightness in your mouth.

Now relax your mouth muscles. Feel the tension drain away from your lips. Feel the warm, comfortable sensation of relaxing.

(Repeat this exercise.)

12. Squint your eyes tightly shut and wrinkle your nose. Hold this tense position. Feel the cramped tightness in your upper face.

Now relax your face muscles. Feel the tension drain away from your eyes and down your nose. Feel the warm, comfortable sensation of relaxing.

(Repeat this exercise.)

13. Raise your eyebrows as high as you can to wrinkle your forehead. Hold this tense position. Feel the cramped tightness in your forehead and scalp.

Now relax your eyebrows. Feel the tension drain from your forehead. Feel the warm, comfortable sensation of relaxing.

(Repeat this exercise.)

After all these exercises, let your whole body relax. Breathe deeply but naturally. Enjoy the sensation of complete relaxation.

EIGHT

Phase-Two Treatment

MAKING THE IMPROVEMENT PERMANENT

I had a call from a colleague and friend: "Andy, I'd like to send you a TMJ patient of mine. Name is Edward Peterson. Man in his fifties—fifty-six to be exact. Came to me with MPD symptoms. Some clicking and retrodiscitis, too. His X-rays showed the condyles pretty high and far back in the joints."

"I made him a repositioning splint to bring the mandible down and forward," my friend went on. "Worked like a charm. He feels just fine, and the clicking goes away. But only as long as he's wearing the splint. As soon as I try to wean him off—even to wearing it just at night—back comes the pain and the clicking. I'm afraid he needs more extensive treatment than I'm prepared to give him. One thing I do know—he doesn't want to wear the splint for the rest of his life, and I can't blame him."

I made an appointment to see Mr. Peterson a week later, and he came with the indispensable splint in his mouth. As with many people his age, his teeth showed a lot of wear and tear. All of them were considerably worn, and he had lost some of his lower molars. The lower jaw overclosed—met the upper jaw at a much higher position than it should have. As a result he had a partly *collapsed* bite, which lacked its full vertical dimension.

When I saw the condition of the teeth, the mystery of the splint was solved. A collapsed bite is quite enough to produce the chewing-muscle fatigue that results in myofascial pain. It can also lead to disk displacement as the high position of the condyles squeezes the disks forward. The splint was in effect making up for his lost and worn-down teeth. It restored the vertical dimension of his bite and helped recapture the disks. As long as he was wearing it, he experienced no pain and no clicking. But as soon as he tried to do without it, even for part of the day, the symptoms returned.

That's the limitation of phase-one treatment for many patients. It can relieve symptoms, but it may not lead to permanent recovery. The basic cause of the disorder—in this case malocclusion—remains. To remedy such basic conditions, it is often necessary to go beyond simple, reversible phase-one therapies to more complicated, nonreversible phase-two procedures.

The simplest remedy I could have provided Ed Peterson was a permanent splint—a new splint rather like the one he already had. It would have been made of tooth-colored plastic over a heavily reinforced metal framework, with stainless steel plugs on the surface at the points of greatest wear. He would have worn it all the time, and it would have lasted several years before wearing out. But that wasn't what he wanted. He hoped that he could return to something like normal, free of his TMJ problems but also free of the splint.

That meant finding some effective form of phase-two treatment for him. It would have been useless to do so before phase-one treatment had relieved his symptoms.

Phase-two procedures, performed on a patient in pain, can unfortunately reinforce the basic conditions that cause the symptoms. In Ed Peterson's case, the splint had made him symptom-free, and it was now possible to choose among the wide variety of phase-two techniques available, from equilibration to orthodontics.

• Equilibration

I have suggested the importance of a *balanced* bite, in which the teeth meet evenly and at the proper angles. If the bite is thrown off balance, so are the muscles, leading to fatigue and pain. Ed Peterson's condition, a *collapsed* bite, was extreme. But even people with a full set of healthy teeth may have an unbalanced bite if the teeth are unequal in height or crooked.

If the problem is not severe, it can sometimes be remedied by a procedure called *equilibration*, a long Latinate word meaning "balance." To achieve equilibration, the dentist selectively grinds and smooths certain "high spots"—areas of individual teeth that stick up too far or meet those in the other jaw at the wrong angle. It is surprising how even minor irregularities can interfere with closing and other normal movements of the jaws. Removal of a little of the hard enamel surfaces of the teeth can thus have a far-reaching effect on their function and can be carried out without doing them any harm.

You've probably encountered equilibration already, at least on a small scale. When a dentist inserts a filling in a tooth or puts a crown over it, that tooth and others nearby must often be equilibrated—ground selectively—to assure a proper relationship with one another. This is a standard procedure in dentistry and, if only a few teeth are involved, should make no basic or irreversible change in the bite.

Following phase-one TMJ treatment, however, much more extensive equilibration may be required, involving many or most of the teeth and making a fundamental change in the bite. This is especially true if a repositioning splint (which changes the relationship of the jaws) has been used. Once the splint has relieved the symptoms, the dentist will first attempt to "walk back" the patient's lower jaw toward its former closing position. Often, however, that process simply causes the symptoms to return. It then becomes necessary to establish a balanced bite with the jaw in the *new* position.

Often the dentist will first do a dry run (literally and figuratively), trying out the intended changes on plaster casts of the teeth before going to work on the teeth themselves. And, while working on the teeth, he or she will undoubtedly check the work as it progresses. Periodically the patient will bite and slide the teeth on sheets of colored wax or paper, showing the main points of contact between the jaws and thus identifying areas that need reducing.

• Restorative Dentistry

Equilibration is a selective process of *subtraction,* by which small portions of enamel are removed from individual teeth. *Addition* is often needed as well, to bring worn or badly positioned teeth into proper working relationships and to replace teeth that are missing. Various dental restorations are used for this purpose.

Whenever possible, the dentist will work from the existing teeth or whatever parts of them are salvageable. The simplest way to restore teeth that are worn, for example, is to build them up with some form of *onlay*. These may be plastic veneers, laminated on the biting surfaces and shaped to create the desired relationship with the teeth in the other jaw. The acrylic materials now available for this purpose are remarkably strong and can last several years. They can also be colored to match the teeth closely, so the restoration is hardly noticeable.

For durability, though, nothing beats the traditional gold. Gold is still widely used for restorations, particularly of back molars, which get heavy wear and are not usually visible. A gold onlay functions like an acrylic one, building up the biting surface.

Sometimes, however, a tooth is too worn or damaged to be restored simply with an onlay. The entire portion above the gum must be covered over with an *artificial crown*, or *cap*. A well-made and well-installed gold crown can last many years. A metallic crown can also be surfaced with ceramic porcelain. This has the advantage of matching the other teeth and is often used for teeth that are highly visible.

To achieve a properly balanced bite, it is important—indeed, often essential—to replace missing teeth. Ed Peterson's lost molars were a major factor in his collapsed bite. But the failure to replace missing teeth can lead to other problems as well.

Teeth are not permanently fixed in one place—their position is stabilized by the teeth next to them and by those in the opposing jaw. When one or more teeth are lost, the other teeth are likely to drift into the space left vacant. Malocclusion can easily result, sometimes leading in turn to TMJ disorders, or making existing ones worse.

The usual method of replacing missing teeth next to sound ones is to make a *bridge*. The "span" of the bridge is made up of one or more artificial teeth attached to a sound *abutment* tooth on one or both sides. The strongest way to attach a bridge is to cover each abutment with a gold or porcelain crown, to which the artificial teeth are soldered.

When many or all of the teeth are missing, partial or complete *dentures* may be necessary. Dentures anchor the artificial teeth in artificial gums, slipped over what remains of the natural ones. It's usually not difficult to create a balanced bite with dentures, which are built from scratch. Sometimes it's possible to position new artificial teeth in an existing base to achieve the desired bite—a procedure called "jumping" the teeth.

In recent years, more and more dentists are using *implantation* techniques to anchor bridgework and dentures firmly in place. The natural gums are opened up surgically and metallic implants are attached permanently to the jawbones. The artificial teeth are attached to the implants by screws, clips, or even magnets. The technique has become even more popular as a result of the happy discovery that the metal titanium becomes naturally bonded (or *integrated*) with bone. Now most implants are titanium.

All these restorative methods make substantial changes, both in the bite and in the other movements of the jaws. Moreover, these changes are usually irreversible. It is therefore essential to proceed with extreme care when trying to use them to resolve TMJ disorders. They should *not* be started until the patient's symptoms have been resolved with phase-one treatment. Otherwise there's a great risk that the procedures will not help but instead will make matters worse, with little or no hope of further remedy.

Furthermore, before restoration can be undertaken, substantial advance work must be done. A complete dental examination must be done and casts made of the jaws. Any tooth decay or gum disease must be treated. Finally, a systematic overall plan for the restoration must be prepared.

In carrying out restoration on TMJ patients, dentists often use a phase-one splint—especially if it's a repositioning splint—as a guide or model. That's precisely what we did for Ed Peterson. We knew he was comfortable only when wearing the splint, which considerably altered the position of his bite. So the splint became a model for restoring his teeth to match the "new" bite.

We literally cut the splint in half, from front to back, so we could work on one side of his mouth at a time. We first made a temporary plastic bridge for the left side of his lower jaw. It not only filled in the gaps left by the missing molars, but also had crowns that built up the worn teeth to a proper height. The biting surfaces were shaped to mesh properly with the upper teeth, the position being dictated by the remaining half-splint on the other side.

Mr. Peterson wore this temporary bridge for a week, until we could be sure that it left him symptom-free. During this time we made minor equilibration changes on the biting surfaces—an easy task in plastic. We then removed the remaining half-splint and made a plastic bridge for that side as well. Both temporary bridges were left in place for about two months, until we were sure that the symptoms wouldn't return.

The temporary bridgework was then replaced with permanent porcelain restorations. But even these were cemented in place only temporarily. They were checked over every three months for a year. Only after we knew that the work was entirely successful did we shift to permanent cement.

• Orthodontics

Maria Leone was feeling much better. A bright and energetic woman of 26, who spoke three languages and worked for a busy import-export company, she had come to me four months before, suffering from persistent earaches. She was also aware of loud clicking, particularly in the right joint, whenever she opened or closed her mouth. Examination revealed disk displacement on the right side. I made her a repositioning splint, designed to bring her mandible downward and forward to recapture the disk. Within a month, her symptoms had subsided.

"So, how are the earaches?" I asked.

"Only one since last time," she replied. "And it was really mild. I think I'm pretty well recovered."

"What about the clicking?"

"Well, there isn't any at all when I wear the splint, and not as much even when I don't." She hesitated a moment. "I do notice it more when I eat. Why is that?"

"Are you by any chance taking out the splint when you eat?"

"Well, yes," she admitted. "I hate the feel of it when I have food in my mouth."

"There's your reason. When you chew without the splint in place, your lower jaw—your mandible—moves back to the old position. The condyles end up too high and too far back, and the disk on the right side shifts forward again."

"I remember now! You warned me something like that might happen. So what's the next step? I'd hate to wear the splint indefinitely."

"To get rid of the splint," I said, "you'll have to do something about the way your teeth mesh together. You see, the way they're positioned now, the upper teeth deflect your lower teeth backward. That causes a bad bite—a malocclusion—with your lower jaw meeting the upper one too far back."

"But couldn't I just get into the habit of biting a little farther forward?"

"By itself, that wouldn't work," I said. "The teeth just wouldn't meet properly. You'd have trouble chewing, and the basic imbalance would be likely to set off more TMJ troubles."

"So does that mean a permanent splint?"

"That's one possibility. But for someone like yourself—relatively young, with sound teeth and healthy gums—there's still another possible solution. And that's orthodontics."

"Orthodontics?" she said doubtfully. "You mean braces? I thought those were just for kids."

"Not at all," I assured her. "Adults get very good results, too. You might at least consult an orthodontist about your condition, before making any decision."

She agreed to this suggestion, and I referred her to a colleague at Mount Sinai. At our next appointment, she reported that she had seen him and that his diagnosis essentially matched mine. Still reluctant about a course of treatment that would probably take up to two years, she had gotten a second opinion on her own, but the advice was the same. She decided to go ahead.

• How Orthodontics Works

Teeth don't just sit there in the jaws. When not restrained by other teeth, they can gradually drift from their proper positions. Too much pressure from neighboring teeth can force them out of line. Furthermore, unless they meet the resistance of other teeth they continue to grow from the gums, not only when they first erupt in childhood but throughout life. Their seemingly stable position results only from a delicate balance of the forces exerted on them by bones and muscles and by one another.

These conditions form the basis of the science—and

art—of *orthodontics* (from Greek words that mean "correcting the teeth"). And orthodontics *does* correct the position of the teeth, through gradual but persistent mechanical pressure.

Contrary to what many people think, orthodontics is not limited to cosmetic "teeth straightening." In fact, orthodontists pay just as much attention, if not more, to assuring an effective and stable occlusion. They know that the working relationship of the jaws is largely determined by the position of the teeth. Thus, their techniques form an important part of the arsenal used for the phase-two treatment of TMJ disorders. For sometimes what is needed to establish the healthful, pain-free function of the joint is to change the position of the teeth to establish a better relationship between the jaws.

• Who Needs Orthodontics?

What most often makes orthodontics necessary for TMJ patients is a situation like Maria Leone's, where a repositioning splint has been used to bring forward the mandible and recapture a displaced disk. The symptoms may be relieved, but the mandible may no longer be able to return to its former position without reviving them. A new bite must be established and stabilized in the position dictated by the splint.

Sometimes restorative dentistry will accomplish this purpose. But for patients like Ms. Leone it usually isn't the best solution. It is better not to put onlays or caps on healthy natural teeth, but to use orthodontics instead to move them into a satisfactory relationship. For example, Maria Leone's condition was a fairly common one. Her teeth—particularly her molars and premolars—were not set at the proper angles, and when she closed her jaws, the lower teeth were driven backward rather than forward. The teeth in both jaws would have to be adjusted so they would meet in a stable, comfortable, and efficient bite at a more forward position.

There are several other types of malocclusion that a splint will not cure, and that may justify orthodontic treatment after phase-one therapy is completed. Controversy still goes on about the relationship between malocclusion and TMJ disorders, but many dentists believe that conditions such as the following can lead to myofascial pain, disk displacement, or both.

- The lower jaw may be smaller than the upper one. In extreme cases, the mandible closes entirely inside the upper jaw, and the teeth hardly meet at all. This *overclosure* puts strain on the muscles and makes them work too hard. It may also lead to disk displacement if the condyles are forced upward in the process.
- The lower jaw may be larger than the upper. This often forces the patient to chew with a sideward-sliding *crossbite*, which fatigues the muscles and stresses the joints.
- The teeth in one jaw may not meet those in the other in an even plane. For instance, when the back teeth meet there may be a gap between the teeth in front—a condition called an *anterior open bite*. Too few teeth end up doing too much work, and the imbalance strains the chewing muscles and loads the joints.
- Misaligned individual teeth may get in the way of a desirable bite and force the jaws to meet in a harmful position. So can teeth that are crowded too close together, spaced too far apart, or drifting into a gap left by a lost tooth.
- The teeth may not be symmetrical from side to side, either in one jaw or in both. As a result the bite becomes lopsided, with some muscles working harder than others.

The imbalance can produce muscle fatigue and pain or shift one or both condyles into positions that squeeze the disks.

Orthodontics can help many such problems. The dental arches of both the lower and upper jaws can be made wider or narrower for a better match in size. Crooked teeth can be straightened. Teeth can be raised or lowered in their sockets so they meet evenly. And the results of treatment can be stabilized so they'll be long-lasting.

But that's a potential drawback as well as an advantage. Like restorative dentistry, orthodontic treatment produces results that are usually irreversible. Consequently it should be undertaken with care and its effects closely monitored both during treatment and afterward—a period that is likely to last for some years.

• Orthodontic Techniques

The basic techniques orthodontists use to shift the teeth and jaws around have been in existence for more than half a century. But the latest methods are less conspicuous, more comfortable, and somewhat quicker. Even so, orthodontics by its nature cannot be a hasty process. In essence, enough mechanical force is applied to move the teeth gradually, steadily, and painlessly. If the force is too strong, it may not only cause discomfort but also do lasting damage to the teeth and gums.

Most orthodontists still find fixed appliances—braces—their most reliable and efficient tools, because they can be controlled so precisely. Traditional braces have been considerably improved in recent years. No longer do metal bands have to be inserted over all the teeth. The brackets through which the bracing wires run can be bonded right onto the tooth surfaces. The brackets themselves are less conspicuous, and now a new, transparent, and even less visible variety is coming into use.

Nonetheless some people will not—or cannot—put up with the visual evidence of treatment. If you are a television anchor, for instance, it may not be professionally advantageous to appear on camera with a mouthful of braces. Such patients may prefer appliances attached entirely inside the teeth. These are virtually invisible, but have the drawbacks of being less comfortable (the tongue is *very* conscious of the intrusion) and of making speech more difficult. They are also a little harder to control and may take a bit longer to get results.

For patients who cannot tolerate even internally attached braces, there are what are called *functional* appliances, which are easily removable and are worn only part of the time. Many orthodontists champion them and maintain that they work just as well as fixed appliances. They do, however, make speech quite difficult while they are worn. And they require the complete cooperation of the patient, who must wear them faithfully for as long as treatment takes.

Actually, there is no single kind of appliance that will suit all conditions, any more than there is a single shoe size that will fit all feet. Most orthodontists use fixed, invisible, and functional appliances alike, basing their choice on the needs of the particular patient.

• Orthodontic Examination and Diagnosis

When Maria Leone returned to the orthodontist for treatment, he made a careful survey of her condition, including a thorough examination and new models of her teeth and jaws. He took color "before" photographs of her full face and profiles. He made standard dental X-rays of her teeth and panoramic views of the whole sweep of her jaws. He also arranged to have a special set of X-rays taken—*cephalometric* ("head-measuring") X-rays that show the entire side of the face, including the relationship of the jaws, on each side.

Following his studies, he discussed various alternatives of treatment with Ms. Leone, and they agreed upon a systematic plan, utilizing fixed appliances, that he estimated would take about eighteen months. This would be followed by at least one year of follow-up stabilization with a removable retaining appliance, plus ongoing examination to make sure the treatment would last.

Nowadays many orthodontists themselves provide phase-one treatment for TMJ disorders and follow it with orthodontic treatment when appropriate. Others, like Ms. Leone's orthodontist, prefer to treat only those TMJ patients whose symptoms have already been stabilized by dentists such as myself. In any event, all symptoms should be under control before phase-two treatment begins. Despite Ms. Leone's understandable impatience, her orthodontist insisted that she remain essentially free of symptoms for at least six weeks before he started inserting appliances.

There are several reasons for such caution. The main reason is that orthodontics is usually irreversible. If orthodontic treatment is undertaken and fails to remedy the TMJ symptoms, it is difficult, if not impossible, to undo.

Furthermore, symptoms such as pain or clicking mean that phase-one treatment has not yet succeeded. The orthodontist has no guidance as to what his own treatment should aim to accomplish. Conversely, successful phase-one treatment provides the orthodontist with an invaluable model for the changes that need to be made. For example, a repositioning splint (like Maria Leone's) that successfully remedies pain and clicking becomes a kind of blueprint for the jaw relationship the orthodontist will work toward.

Incidentally, if you are looking for a capable orthodontist (for a TMJ disorder or some other problem), here are some of the things to look for. He or she should be a member of the American Association of Orthodontists. You should be given a thorough examination, including a complete medical and dental history. Models will be cast from your jaws, and your face will be photographed. Extensive X-rays, including panoramic and cephalometric views, will be taken.

Following the examination, the orthodontist should be able to explain the diagnosis clearly to you and should provide you a fairly precise plan of treatment, specifying the aims to be achieved, the procedures to be used, and the timetable to be followed (orthodontics takes a while).

If you should happen to consult the orthodontist while you are suffering pain or other symptoms, be wary if he or she proposes to begin immediate orthodontic treatment "to make you feel better." And *never* hesitate to get a second opinion. Orthodontics is time-consuming and expensive, and should not be entered into lightly.

• The Course of Treatment

Maria Leone's treatment followed a rather typical orthodontic course. It was carried out in several stages and made use of the repositioning splint itself. Earlier I described how I cut such a splint apart and left half of it in place while restoring the teeth on the other side. Orthodontists sometimes do much the same thing.

In this case, the orthodontist started by bonding braces on both the upper and lower teeth. Next, while Ms. Leone continued to wear her splint, he applied pressure to the bracing wires running through the brackets, so that all the teeth would be level, with none misaligned in relation to the others. This process took several weeks.

He then cut away part of the splint to uncover just a few of the upper teeth. He applied pressure to move these teeth, plus the lower ones that faced them, to the desired positions. When this first move was completed he cut away more of the splint, exposing a second group of teeth. Again, pressure was applied to move that group. The same procedure was used until all the teeth were properly positioned. The jaws then met naturally in the same relationship as that established by the splint.

The entire treatment, as planned, took about a year and a half. The braces were then removed. A little equilibration—selective grinding—was needed to adjust the meshing of the tooth surfaces. (In some cases, especially those in which teeth have been lost, orthodontic treatment must be accompanied or followed by substantial restorative dentistry.)

To stabilize the changes that had been made, a plastic retainer, molded to the inside of the upper jaw, was inserted. Maria Leone wore this all the time, except when she ate, for six months, and then wore it only at night for a year more. Some patients, especially those who clench or grind their teeth, must be fitted with a retainer that is also a flat-plane splint, to protect the biting surfaces. They must wear it, at least at night, indefinitely.

The orthodontist examined Ms. Leone at monthly intervals for the first six months and at three-month intervals for the next six months. She now returns every six months to make sure all is well.

I, too, have been monitoring her progress and its effect on the joints. The orthodontic treatment essentially made lasting what the repositioning splint had accomplished temporarily. It moved the condyles slightly forward and downward, so they would retain a proper relationship with the disks. During treatment and afterward, she remained virtually free of TMJ symptoms.

• Can Orthodontics Do Harm?

Orthodontic treatment can and does make substantial changes in the relationship of the jaws. The question naturally arises: Is there any risk that such treatment will affect the joints in a harmful way? Can it, in fact, lead to TMJ disorders? The answer is usually no, but occasionally yes. Most orthodontists have become very sensitive to joint problems and are careful to assure that the condyles are properly placed when treatment is complete.

There are two possible exceptions. The first is an effort to remedy *prognathism,* a condition in which the lower teeth jut out in front of the upper ones, creating the visual effect of a "bulldog chin." If the lower teeth and jaw are simply pulled backward, the condyles may be pulled back as well and can end up pressing into the backs of the joints. Inflammation and pain are a likely result.

The second possible exception is an effort to change outwardly protruding upper front teeth. This is a very common condition, and orthodontic treatment can easily move the teeth back to a much better-looking alignment. But if the teeth are simply pivoted backward, without moving their roots, they may end up at too upright an angle in the upper jaw. Then the lower front teeth, closing against the backs of the upper ones, may force the whole lower jaw back to a new position. Movement of the jaw is likely to be restricted, and joint inflammation and muscular pain can result.

These problems really shouldn't come up, but I tell prospective patients about them to explain why an orthodontist must often specify treatment that goes much further than simply "straightening the teeth."

• The Limits of Phase-Two Treatment

There are some conditions that neither restorative dentistry nor orthodontics can cure. In some cases, such as osteoarthritis of the joint, treatment can maintain the patient in reasonable comfort but cannot undo the damage. Furthermore, some structural defects of the jaws are far too severe to be remedied by these kinds of treatment. For these patients the only alternative may be surgery—as I will explain in the next chapter.

NINE

Surgery

WHEN NOTHING ELSE WILL WORK

After seven years of almost constant pain, Laurel Mannes was at the end of her endurance. Every day she felt as if a red-hot spike were being rammed through the top of her skull, and her face hurt so much she couldn't bear to smile. Opening her mouth caused her such agony that she could barely eat or talk. She had been to many doctors and had been subjected to many treatments and drugs, but nothing gave her lasting relief. It was all she could do to hold onto her job as a graphic designer. The stress of publication deadlines seemed to make her physical problems worse.

Her trouble had begun with a serious automobile accident when she was in college. A drunken driver demolished her car and sent her to the hospital with severe neck injuries. Eventually, after surgery on two fractured vertebrae, she seemed to recover and thought she was completely healed. Then she began to suffer the increasingly severe pains in her head, face, and jaw.

The physicians in charge of her rehabilitation were baffled. Like many of the other doctors and chiropractors she was to consult over the years, they thought the pains might be psychological in origin. They prescribed pain relievers and anti-inflammatory drugs and administered physical therapy of various kinds, but the pain just got worse.

Eventually one doctor did diagnose that she was suffering from a TMJ disorder, caused—or at least triggered—by the trauma of her accident. But he, too, gave her little more than drugs to relieve her pain and tried to persuade her the problem was something she would just have to live with. That idea was enough to make her contemplate suicide.

But having discovered that her problem was likely to be a TMJ disorder, she began to look for help from practitioners in that field. A friend gave her the name of an oral surgeon at Mount Sinai. He gave her a complete examination, including the special X-rays called arthrograms.

The evidence seemed fairly plain. During the seven years since her accident, her right TMJ had badly deteriorated. The original trauma had apparently caused dislocation of its articular disk, throwing her bite out of balance.

Moreover, without proper cushioning from the disk she had developed osteoarthritis in the joint; the condyle had become eroded on top and had developed an abnormal growth, called an *osteophyte*, in front (see Figure 15). The arthrograms showed a characteristic change in the shape of the condyle, from a rounded knob to a flattened anvil.

These structural changes produced inflammatory pain in the joint. This led in turn to "guarding" in the chewing muscles—an effort to limit the painful movement. The joint pain and the muscle guarding were what made it difficult for her to open her mouth. The extra strain on the muscles caused fatigue and spasms in them as well, accounting for the pain in her head and face.

The oral surgeon concluded that surgery on the joint

offered the best chance of relieving these symptoms. But he first wanted to make sure that they could not be helped with less drastic treatment, so he referred her to me for evaluation. After reviewing his findings and making my own examination, I agreed with his diagnosis. Laurel Mannes met what I consider three basic criteria for TMJ surgery:

- The disorder was *severe*, causing extreme debility. Her situation was desperate, in both a physical and emotional sense.
- The disorder was *structural.* It arose from abnormalities in the joint itself: a dislocated disk that had led to osteoarthritis.
- Other treatment had *failed*, and there was no reasonable alternative. Medications gave her little relief. I made a splint for her to help reduce the inflammation, but the disk was too far dislocated to be recaptured in that way. Furthermore, there was nothing I could do to remedy the changes in the bone.

• Disk Plication

The surgery to be performed on Laurel Mannes was the most common type for TMJ disorders, (*disk plication*, literally a "tying of the disk"). The disk, which has slipped forward off the condyle, is pulled back onto it and sutured (sewed) in place. There is, of course, more to the process than that, as we will see.

Surgery on the TMJ has become more common during the last ten years or so; earlier efforts were often unsuccessful. Greater knowledge of how the joint works, plus better diagnostic techniques, have now given us a clearer idea of the conditions surgery can help. Disk plication now produces significant improvement for about 80 per cent of the patients who undergo it. And the results seem to last, although the procedure has not been in use long enough for anyone to be completely sure of its long-term consequences.

I must emphasize that surgery is not a *substitute* for other treatment, either phase one or phase two. It is the treatment of last resort, either when other methods have already failed or when they plainly won't work. Moreover, it must often settle for something short of a complete and perfect cure. Rather, it aims for significant improvement in the patient's comfort and ability to function.

The operation on Laura Mannes' right TMJ provides a clear picture of the successive steps of disk plication. She came into the hospital the night before, to be ready for surgery first thing in the morning. She had already been examined by her regular internist, and at the hospital was also given a thorough physical examination, including X-rays, urine and blood tests, and consultation with the anesthesiologist, to make sure there were no conditions that would interfere with surgery.

Preparation for the operation itself was fairly simple. First, she was given a sedative to diminish any apprehension she might feel. Most of her hair was enclosed in what was essentially a plastic shower cap, and the area of her cheek in front of her ear was swabbed with antiseptic.

For most surgery, the whole area has to be shaved of hair, but for this kind of operation, such shaving is kept to a minimum. Only a little hair, right at the hairline in front of the ear, is removed, and the lock immediately above is left untouched, so it can be pulled over the shaven area until the hair grows back. As in all surgery involving the face, every effort is devoted toward making the work as inconspicuous as possible.

In the operating room Ms. Mannes was quickly given general anesthesia, so she was completely unconscious throughout the operation. Local anesthesia is theoretically feasible for this kind of surgery, but it is seldom used, since the patient's head must be kept completely immobile.

The surgeon made a small incision, a little less than two inches in length (Figure 20), directly in front of the ear, where a natural crease in the skin would tend to hide the scar. He also shaped the incision into shallow scallops, joined end to end, to avoid the greater conspicuousness of a straight-line scar. From the top he extended the incision obliquely forward for another inch or so. This part would become hidden under the hairline.

His choice of location for the incision was practical as well as aesthetic. Happily, the tissues underneath are relatively free of nerves and blood vessels, which should be left undisturbed as much as possible.

The flap of skin within the V-shaped cut was then

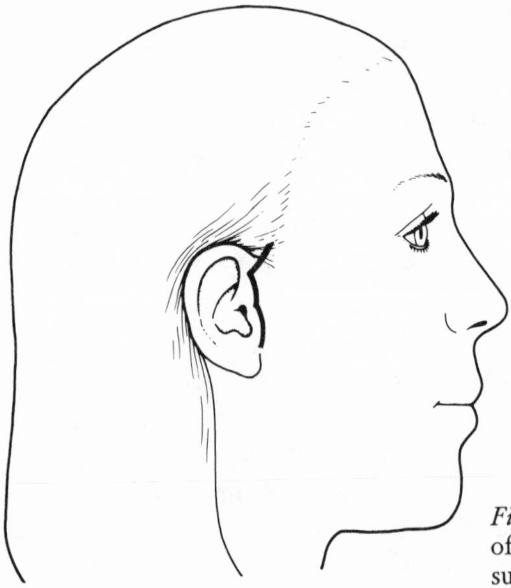

Figure 20. Typical line of incision for joint surgery, to minimize visibility of scar.

pulled back, revealing a portion of the temporalis fascia where it passed under the arch of the cheekbone. The surgeon made an incision lengthwise and pulled the tissue back like a pair of curtains on either side of the incision. This exposed the capsule around the joint. A short horizontal cut then opened up the joint itself.

As often happens, the problems there proved to be even more severe than the X-ray evidence had suggested. The disk was not only displaced in front of the condyle; it was partly torn from its connection to the retrodiscal tissue and was essentially free-floating. The top of the condyle was worn down, and there was an osteophyte on its front edge, as the X-rays had shown. But in addition, the surface was pitted and furrowed. The possible cause was repeated treatment with steroid injections, which can erode cartilage and bone tissue.

So, before he could proceed to fastening the disk back in place, the surgeon had to reshape the condyle into a smooth, even knob. He literally filed down the surface, using a machine-driven file. In the process he also removed the osteophyte growth.

He then gently pulled the disk back over the condyle. Fortunately it was not badly damaged, and there was a good chance that it could be restored to its proper function. Sometimes the disk turns out to be perforated—torn or worn through. In these instances, the perforation can sometimes be repaired by sewing it shut. But some surgeons prefer to remove a perforated disk entirely, replacing it with a piece of pliable plastic. This surgeon chose not to do that, mainly because such replacements have a rather poor record for long-term durability. At present there is no reliable substitute for the living tissue, even if it is damaged.

Before attempting to suture the disk back on top of the condyle, he cut a small, wedge-shaped piece from the outer edge of the retrodiscal tissue, where it had torn away from the disk. He did so for two reasons. First, when the disk is dislocated forward, the retrodiscal tissue gets permanently stretched and will no longer hold the disk in place even if the tear is repaired. Second, the displacement of the disk is usually not only forward but inward. Cutting a triangular wedge from the outer edge of the retrodiscal tissue, and then suturing the disk, to it pulls the disk both backward and outward, so it ends up in the proper position right on top of the condyle.

The surgeon also "cleaned" the spaces above and below the disk. Sometimes, when the disk is displaced or damaged, blood vessels in the surrounding tissues are ruptured. The blood then clots and forms fibrous tissues, similar to scar tissue, in the joint spaces. These fibrous tissues can form connections (called *adhesions*) between the disk and the temporal bones. These may prevent the disk from moving properly with the condyle when the jaw opens. Some experts believe that such adhesions are a major cause of reduced jaw movement. In any event, it is generally agreed that if present they should be removed during the operation.

To stabilize the disk further, the surgeon sutured its outer edge to ligament tissue on the side of the condyle. He then filed away a little of the articular eminence of the temporal bone along which the condyle and the disk slide when the jaw opens fully.

This last procedure is not unusual, but there are two schools of thought about it. Some surgeons prefer not to disturb the bone surfaces at all. Others believe that providing additional space for the disk between the condyle and the eminence will make opening the jaw easier and smoother and will help prevent the disk from becoming dislocated again.

The surgeon checked his work by manually opening

and closing the mandible, to make sure that the disk was in the right location at every stage of movement. Then he sutured the incisions in the joint capsule, the temporalis fascia, and the skin. He used especially fine sutures, the kind employed for eye surgery, to close the incision through the skin, so they would leave no marks when they were removed. Finally he placed a temporary pressure bandage over the area to minimize swelling.

The operation took about an hour and a half. Ms. Mannes was then taken to the recovery room to regain consciousness and remained in the hospital overnight. Next morning the bandage was removed and she was released. Three days later she went to the surgeon's office to have the stitches in her skin removed. The scar was already hardly noticeable, and, when healing was complete, it became invisible.

For a few days the area remained tender and a little swollen, simply from the operation. She was given mild anti-inflammatory medications, which minimized her discomfort. She also stuck to a soft diet for about three weeks, so as not to "load" the joint with heavy chewing, then gradually went back to ordinary food over the following month.

A week or so after the operation, the tenderness and swelling had subsided enough so she could begin a program of physical therapy. This is an important part of the healing process. I have mentioned that bleeding leads to the formation of fibrous scar tissue and adhesions. During the operation, bleeding is kept to a minimum, but a little is inevitable. The gentle, controlled exercises provided during physical therapy reduce the formation of scar tissue and help prevent it from stiffening the joint and undoing the benefits of surgery.

For Laurel Mannes, the benefits were almost immediately apparent. Within a week the agonizing muscular pains in her head and face disappeared. She might not be able to open her mouth into a wide yawn, but at least she could eat and speak normally. She returned to work, and her colleagues weren't even aware of the surgery—except for the evident change in her morale. For the first time in years she felt free—free of pain, free of useless treatments, free to live an ordinary life. As she put it, "I felt like I had broken out of prison."

The entire healing process took a little over two months. During this time, I had her continue using the splint I had made for her, at least at night, to keep the pressure on the joint to a minimum. She still wears it occasionally, when stress or a change in the weather produces a slight ache in the joint. But most of the time, some three years after the operation, she remains virtually symptom-free.

In one respect, Laurel Mannes' cases was a simple one. The original cause of her disorder was an accident, and once she was correctly diagnosed and surgery was performed, her difficulties were largely over. Sometimes, even after surgery, further treatment is required—to break a grinding habit, say, or remedy malocclusion. Also, the surgery may itself change the pattern of the bite, making phase-two treatment necessary to adjust the teeth.

It must be acknowledged that all such stories don't end happily. For from 10 to 20 percent of all patients, disk-plication surgery doesn't produce satisfactory results. For some there is no significant improvement in the range of movement of the lower jaw—they still can't open it normally. Others experience a temporary improvement (just cutting through the small nerves in the capsule causes the joint to go numb for a while), but the pain returns when the nerves regenerate. And if the disk is in such poor condition that it must be removed, no artificial replacement is likely to last permanently.

It is up to the surgeon to warn prospective patients about these limitations as part of obtaining the patient's "informed consent." The surgeon should also make the patient aware of the rare but possible complications that can follow surgery. If, for example, part of the facial nerve is accidentally severed, the patient may be left with a condition called *Bell's palsy*. The eyelid droops, yet cannot be fully closed; the forehead can't be wrinkled; the side of the face is numb, temporarily or permanently. This very seldom happens, but scattered instances have been reported.

There is also very slight, but real, risk in *any* operation involving general anesthesia, whether TMJ surgery or having an appendix removed. That's why the operation must be performed in a hospital, with an anesthesiologist present.

If you have a severe TMJ disorder and contemplate surgery, the chances are that you will be referred to an oral surgeon by the dentist treating you. There are, though, some credentials you should look for. He or she should be *board-certified* by the American Association of Oral and Maxillofacial Surgeons. Do not be shy about asking.

And don't hesitate to ask other questions, either. Here are a few:

- Where do you perform this kind of surgery?

(A major hospital or medical center is preferable to a small, proprietary hospital.)

- How often do you perform it?

(There's no absolute rule of thumb, but if the answer is fewer than four or five a year, the surgeon may not have enough experience or may be rusty.)

- What is your experience with cases like mine? What is my outlook?

(The surgeon should be able to estimate the chances of success.)

Finally, in any procedure as serious as surgery, I can't stress enough that a second opinion is well worth the time, trouble, and expense.

• Arthroscopic Surgery

In very recent years, a new technique has appeared that, in some cases, obviates the need for "open-joint" TMJ surgery. Called *arthroscopic* surgery, the technique was first developed in Japan and is already much used for surgery on knee joints. Its application to the much smaller TMJ used to be rare but is rapidly gaining in popularity.

Arthroscopic surgery is performed with the assistance of an *arthroscope* (literally, "something that looks into the joint"). It is basically a miniature microscope that looks rather like a hypodermic syringe. At the end of the "needle" is a tiny magnifying lens, surrounded by optical fibers that conduct light to the area being viewed.

This apparatus enters the joint through a cylindrical metal sheath, which itself has such a small diameter—no more than two-and-a-half millimeters—that it can be inserted by making a puncture through the skin and other soft tissues. The puncture wound requires no sutures and leaves almost no mark behind it. There is nonetheless enough room in the sheath for a salt-water solution to be pumped through it even when the arthroscope is in place, to bathe and open up the joint space.

The image can be viewed directly by the eye, but a special video camera is generally used instead. This enlarges and projects the image (in full color) on a screen. Often it is recorded on videotape at the same time.

The arthroscope gives a highly detailed, well-defined view of the joint structures. It clearly reveals a disk that is displaced forward and retrodiscal tissue that has been pulled forward over the condyle. It shows a tear or perforation of the disc and degenerative changes from osteoarthritis. And it also shows inflammation of the soft tissues and any scar tissue or adhesions that may have formed.

Arthroscopy by itself is potentially very valuable as a diagnostic tool. It provides more direct evidence of capsulitis, retrodiscitis, and disk displacement than any other imaging technique. But it may also be used for *treatment*—arthroscopic *surgery*. A second cylindrical sheath is inserted into the joint space a short distance from the first. Through it can be passed miniature surgical instruments, such as blunt-ended probes, curettes for scraping, scalpels, even forceps and scissors. The surgery is viewed through the arthroscope as it proceeds. But the instruments are very small, the working space is very small, and the number of procedures possible is at present limited.

For example, surgeons are still working to come up with a way to perform the kind of disk plication described earlier. And as yet there's no way of using arthroscopic surgery to repair a torn or perforated disk. The technique is most often used to remove pieces of scar tissue and adhesions. These can be rubbed off the joint tissues with a probe, scraped off with a curette, pulled off with forceps, cut off with a scalpel or scissors, and then flushed away with the irrigating solution.

The surgeons who perform this procedure believe that, for certain patients, clearing away these fibrous materials can be very effective. In particular, they feel that disk displacement is often caused, or at least made worse, by adhesions between the disk and the temporal bone, which cause the disk to "hang up" rather than slide smoothly. In any event, some patients report significant relief from their symptoms after arthroscopy has "opened up" the joint.

Like open-joint surgery, arthroscopic surgery is usually

performed under general anesthesia, but since it is less invasive recovery is faster and easier. A pressure bandage is applied for a few hours to keep down bleeding, but there are no stitches, and the small punctures are simply covered with a Band-Aid until they heal.

There may be some swelling and tenderness for a day or two; they are treated with anti-inflammatory medications and the like. But the symptoms are less severe and go away faster than those following open-joint surgery. Physical therapy begins the day after the operation, to prevent the formation of new scar tissue.

Arthroscopic surgery has reached a state where it is much more than simply experimental. For some patients it already obviates the need for open-joint surgery. And even when it does not succeed and open-joint surgery is necessary, the videotaped record allows the surgeon to plan the operation with greater precision.

At present, arthroscopic surgery is the subject of a great deal of research, and substantial advances in its usefulness are likely. For example, at least one surgeon has come up with a possible substitution for disk plication. Instead of removing a piece of the retrodiscal tissue and sewing the disk to what remains, he shrinks the retrodiscal tissue with high heat so that it pulls the disk back in place.

Complications are somewhat less likely with arthroscopic surgery. Some of them are the same as those with open-joint procedures. The risks resulting from general anesthesia are the same. There is also a very slight danger of damaging a nerve or of causing problems with hearing.

In addition, there are some risks associated specifically with arthroscopy. There's a slight chance that the needle-like end of the arthroscope or one of the fine surgical instruments will break off in the joint, will hit a blood vessel, or even perforate the inside of the joint and enter the skull cavity and the brain. Although these risks are quite remote, informed consent requires that the patient be aware of them. The patient must also agree in advance to let the surgeon proceed immediately to open-joint surgery to remedy any such complications should they arise.

Surgeons who perform arthroscopic surgery are still relatively few in number. If you need a referral, request information from the International Study Group for TMJ Arthroscopy (address in the Appendix).

• Orthognathic Surgery

Some conditions call for treatment more drastic than either open-joint or arthroscopic surgery. These are basic defects in the bones of the jaws that sometimes result from trauma but more often are hereditary. Relatively mild instances can sometimes be remedied with restorative dentistry or orthodontics, but severe ones may require *orthognathic* ("jaw-correcting") *surgery.*

Four of these conditions are particularly associated with TMJ disorders:

- The mandible is too large in comparison with the upper jaw. As a result, the mandible is said to be *prognathic*, or jutting forward, more popularly described as "bulldog chin." By itself, this doesn't necessarily cause a TMJ disorder. However, some patients, and some dentists or orthodontists who should know better, try to push the teeth into a normal bite. The usual result, as the teeth mesh together, is for the mandible to be pushed backward, so that each condyle presses against the back of its fossa. This causes retrodiscitis and often leads to disk displacement as well.
- The mandible is too small in comparison with the upper jaw. In moderately severe cases, this condition is called *retrognathia*, or "backward jaw"; in really severe

ones, it is called *micrognathia*, or "small jaw." The visual effect is of a receded, "weak" chin. Sometimes the upper teeth close entirely over those in the short and narrow mandible, producing what looks like a collapsed bite. To make matters worse, many people try to minimize the effect by consciously thrusting the lower jaw forward. In any event, the chewing muscles are thrown badly off balance and the eventual result is myofascial pain dysfunction (MPD).

• The bones that form the upper jaw grow downward too much, producing what is called *long-face syndrome*. This is a fairly common condition with several adverse effects. The whole face appears to be long and narrow. The line of the lips is high, so the smile reveals much of the upper gum. Sometimes the lips can't be completely closed at all, and the chin is flattened by muscles trying to bring the lips together. More serious, the mandible is moved to a less efficient position by the overly deep upper jaw, and the chewing muscles are forced to work harder; in fact, they never achieve a completely relaxed state. The result is fatigue and myofascial pain.

• The bones on one side are larger (or smaller) than those on the other, producing *asymmetry*. The face often looks lopsided, and the mandible slides sidewise as it opens. Again, the muscles are out of balance, resulting in myofascial pain.

When these conditions are severe, they can seldom be remedied with a splint, by restorative dentistry, or by orthodontics. The bones themselves must often be reshaped, which requires surgery. The three surgical procedures used for the purpose can be performed entirely from within the mouth, so they leave no visible scars:

• To remedy prognathism, the mandible can be *short-*

ened. On each side, the part called the *ramus,* which extends upward behind the teeth, is cut so that the part containing the condyle is separated from the rest. Then either some of the bone is cut away, or the two pieces are simply made to overlap (this part of the jawbone is relatively thin and flat). The pieces may be wired together, but the regrowth of bone between them is what bonds them permanently.

In executing this procedure, and all the others, the surgeon must make sure that the new relationship of the jaws and teeth results in a proper position for the condyle in the joint.

• To remedy retrognathism, the mandible can be *lengthened.* The procedure most often used now is called a *sagittal split.* The jawbone is cut, just behind the teeth on each side, but not straight through. Instead, two shallow parallel cuts are made an inch or so apart, one on the inside and the other on the outside. The bone is then sliced apart lengthwise between the cuts so that the pieces form what a carpenter would call a lap joint. The front of the mandible is slid forward, so a partial overlap remains. In healing, not only do the pieces knit together but new bone grows to fill in the depressions beside the overlap.

This procedure can be combined with others to reshape a micrognathic jaw. If the mandible is too narrow, segments can be cut apart and reassembled in a wider arch. And the chin can be built up at the same time by cutting off its point at a diagonal angle, then sliding the piece slightly forward and upward.

• To remedy the long-face syndrome, the bones above the upper jaw can be *reduced in depth.* The bones are cut through horizontally, across the whole width of the jaw, and excess structure is removed before the two pieces are drawn back together. To assure a proper TMJ relationship, it is sometimes necessary to reshape the lower jaw as well, shortening it vertically or lengthening it horizontally by the procedures described above.

Asymmetries in the bones of the jaws are remedied by using the same methods, often in combination. One of our patients, for example, had a mandible that was considerably deeper on one side than the other. The structure of the upper jaw had adjusted to compensate, and so the line of her teeth was tilted from one side to the other, instead of being horizontal. As a result, not only was her face lopsided, but she developed severe pain in the unbalanced chewing muscles as well.

Surgery required reducing the size of the mandible on one side and increasing it on the other. But it was also necessary to make the upper jaw horizontal, by cutting it loose from the rest of the cranium and removing some of the bone on one side before reattaching it.

Orthognathic surgery is obviously a more intrusive process than disk plication in the joint. The procedures must be very carefully planned in advance, often in collaboration with the referring dentist and an orthodontist. They require intensive X-ray studies and are usually tried out on casts of the patient's jaws before they are performed on the patient.

The possible complications of this kind of surgery are about the same as those of disk plication, except that the sagittal split comes quite close to a nerve that registers sensation in the chin, lower teeth, and lower lip. There's a slight risk that, if the nerve is irritated or cut, numbness in those areas could result.

Recovery from such surgery is longer and more complicated than from simpler procedures. The jaws usually have to be immobilized by wiring them together until the bones begin to knit. Surgeons have reduced this period by using temporary metal plates to join the bone segments. These have to be removed later in a second operation. In any event, the patient ordinarily has to stick to a soft diet for at least two months to avoid putting too much pressure on the jaws as they heal.

Orthognathic surgery can have several benefits for appropriate patients. Most important, of course, are the improvement in functioning and the relief of TMJ symptoms. Almost as important, for many patients, is the improvement in their appearance.

The conditions I've described often *harm* appearance, in subtle but undeniable ways. A prognathic jaw, for instance, makes a person seem aggressive and stubborn. A retrognathic jaw looks "weak." The low-slung jaw and slightly open lips of the long-face syndrome suggest dullness and stupidity. Remedying these problems often results in a dramatic and positive change in patients' perception of themselves. Looking better actually helps them feel better.

TEN

WHAT WILL IT COST—AND WHO PAYS?

The first question most patients ask me is "What can you do to help me?" The second is "What will treatment cost?" If they don't ask I tell them, because it's something they should know, in advance. And there's one more question they should also know the answer to: "Can I pay for treatment through insurance?"

Treatment for TMJ disorders is expensive. It requires the skill and attention of highly trained professionals—very often a team of them—working over an extended period. Some of these professionals, such as oral surgeons and orthodontists, may charge a single fixed fee for their services. Others, including dentists like myself, charge fees for individual patient visits and specific procedures and may find it difficult to estimate total treatment costs. Nonetheless, you should discuss costs with the dentist or other practitioner, fully and frankly, *before* treatment begins, to be aware of their likely range and to avoid misunderstandings.

• Relative Costs of Treatment

Treatment costs vary widely from patient to patient, from

doctor to doctor, and from one part of the country to another. Here I'll give at least a range of costs for various kinds of treatment and show how they relate to one another.

A basic TMJ examination of the kind described in Chapter 4 would range anywhere from about $75 to $250. This would include a dental and medical history, a physical examination, casts of the jaws, and an opinion or diagnosis. It would not, however, include X-rays or other imaging techniques, which can run up the diagnostic costs considerably. Some practitioners include X-rays and other diagnostic tests in their consultation; their basic fee would be higher than what I have indicated.

X-rays of the joints, of the kind that can be taken in the dentist's office, would range from $75 to $150. There would be comparable charges for panoramic (Panorex) or cephalometric X-rays.

The selectively focused X-rays called tomograms usually require the special facilities of a medical radiologist. They would cost from $200 to $350 per set. Specialized equipment is also needed for arthrograms, which are used to diagnose a displaced disk. They are often taken on one side only and cost about $250 to $350 per side.

CT scans also require special radiological facilities. Their cost would range from about $350 to $450. The availability of magnetic resonance imaging is now somewhat limited. Its cost would run from $750 to $850 but is expected to drop as the technique becomes more widely used.

One of the most common therapies for TMJ disorders is a flat-plane or repositioning splint. It is made from casts of the patient's jaws, either in the dentist's own office or in a dental laboratory. In either case, the dentist will undoubtedly make adjustments, both when inserting the appliance and on follow-up visits. Some dentists charge a fee for making and inserting the splint and additional fees for the follow-ups. These will range quite widely: $400 to $1200 for making and inserting the splint and $50 to $150 for each of the follow-ups, depending on the time spent and the procedures used. Some dentists charge a flat fee for the whole course of splint therapy of about $1000 to $2000.

Incidentally, if the splint is lost or broken, replacing or repairing it is likely to cost almost as much as the original, since the amount of work is roughly the same.

Phase-one treatment often includes physical therapy, biofeedback therapy, psychological therapy, or some combination of them. Some dentists offer these therapies in their own offices and include them in the overall fee. Usually, however, they are provided separately. Physical therapy would cost about $65 to $100 per session. Biofeedback training would range from $75 to $150 per session. It's hard to estimate the total number of sessions; it varies from patient to patient. As a rough rule of thumb, biofeedback requires about ten sessions for mastery.

Other psychological treatment varies widely in cost, depending on who is providing it. The rate of a social worker might be $65 to $75 per hour, while that of a clinical psychologist or psychotherapist might be $75 to $125 or more. This kind of treatment is open-ended—there's no general rule about how many sessions are "enough."

The cost of phase-two restorative dentistry will vary widely, depending on the extent of the work to be done. Equilibration might require one visit or several, and its cost might range from $100 to $500. Crowns and bridges would cost from $500 to $1000 per tooth, multiplied by the number of teeth involved. A partial denture would range anywhere from $600 to $2000; a complete set would be $1200 to $3000.

Orthodontists usually charge a flat fee for a complete course of treatment that would range from $3000 to $5000, with some further variation according to the complexity of the task. Oral surgeons also charge a flat fee for an operation and its follow-up visits. For joint surgery on one side, the fee would be about $3500 to $6000. For orthognathic surgery it would range from $5500 to $9000—or even higher, depending on the complexity of the operation.

However, the costs of surgery go far beyond the surgeon's fee. A hospital stay of about two days is required, at several hundred dollars a day. An anesthesiologist must be present. Also, either your regular doctor or some other internist must examine you beforehand to clear you for surgery. There may be additional hospital charges for lab tests, X-rays, and medications as well. Finally, surgery often requires a series of physical therapy treatments afterward.

• Cutting Costs—Clinics and Other Alternatives

Treatment for TMJ disorders, especially if phase-two treatment or surgery is involved, can be for many patients a financial burden too heavy to bear. There are a few ways in which costs can be reduced.

Perhaps the simplest and most practical, at least for patients located near a major university or in a metropolitan center, is a teaching clinic such as our TMJ clinic at Mount Sinai in New York City. Treatment is provided by dental residents, or by dentists engaged in postgraduate training, under the supervision of experienced professionals. Such clinics may provide a wide range of services, from TMJ therapy to orthodontics and surgery. Quality of treatment is usually very high, and the cost is usually under the prevailing rates in the area.

But a clinic is not a private office. Patients may have to sacrifice the one-to-one relationship with a particular practitioner. They must fit their own schedule to that of the clinic, which may be open only at certain hours on certain days. And they are likely to do a lot of waiting—waiting for an appointment, waiting to be treated, even waiting to make payment to the clinic cashier.

Certain employment categories entitle patients to reduced rates or even free treatment. Members of the armed forces and some federal workers (from the president on down) can be treated in federal hospitals. Veterans can find dental as well as medical treatment through the VA health system. Employees of universities and medical centers may enjoy reduced rates at institutions that include dental schools or departments.

In certain very limited circumstances, TMJ treatment may be available through Medicare or Medicaid. Medicare may sometimes pay for phase-one treatment, but probably not for phase two. Medicaid is available only to patients with little or no resources. Its fees are fixed and limited, and few private practitioners can afford to accept them. Medicaid patients with TMJ disorders may be able to find treatment in one of the clinics mentioned above. Extended, expensive treatments, such as phase-two procedures, are likely to require authorization in advance.

More and more people are now trying to control their medical costs by joining a health maintenance organization (HMO). An HMO is supposed to provide all medical and dental treatment at a fixed monthly fee, but many of these programs specifically exclude treatment for TMJ disorders. If you're thinking of joining an HMO, better check in advance.

• What about Insurance?

Many people in this country, especially those who are regularly employed, have some form of medical insurance. A sizable proportion have both basic insurance, of which the Blue Cross and Blue Shield programs are the best known, and major medical insurance to protect against the risk of really big expenses. A considerably smaller number have dental insurance as well.

You might think that either medical insurance or dental insurance or both would cover the treatment of TMJ disorders. Unfortunately, the situation is more complicated than that—much more complicated.

There are two main reasons. First, the diagnosis and treatment of TMJ disorders are a relatively recent development, even though the disorders themselves are not. A wide range of techniques is used, and few standard procedures apply to all patients. Thus the insurance carriers face the same difficulties they do with any new procedures. That is, the costs for treating TMJ disorders were not figured into the formulas under which risks and premiums were calculated, and claims thus represent an alarming and unexpected expense. Only recently, and somewhat reluctantly, have insurance companies begun to adjust to the change.

The second reason has to do with the particular location of the disorders and the manner in which they are treated. The joints connect the bones that hold the teeth. Furthermore, their disorders are often related to problems with the teeth, such as malocclusion, grinding, and clenching. Treatment has therefore most often been provided by dentists, using dental techniques such as splints, restoration, orthodontics, and oral surgery.

On the other hand, TMJ disorders are not basically

dental problems, any more than disorders of the elbows or knees are. The result has been confusion and controversy. Many medical insurers have tried to characterize TMJ disorders as dental problems, not covered by medical insurance. Dental carriers have done the reverse, calling them medical problems, not covered by dental insurance. The patient is of course left out in the cold, with no one willing to pay.

In 1982, the American Dental Association tried to resolve the controversy with a proposal that phase-one procedures be considered medical treatment and phase-two procedures dental. There is some logic to this. Phase-one treatment attempts to relieve physical symptoms, and many of its methods (heat and cold, anti-inflammatory medications, electrical stimulation, and so on) are exactly the same as those used to treat other musculoskeletal disorders. Phase-two treatment, by contrast, is customarily used to relieve dental problems, regardless of whether or not TMJ disorders are involved.

Some insurance companies now appear disposed to accept this rule of thumb. It has also been mandated by the legislature of at least one state, Minnesota, for all medical policies issued in that state. But the solution is not entirely satisfactory from the patient's point of view. For one thing, relatively few people carry dental insurance. More important, TMJ disorders really are medical problems, as any sufferer from MPD or a dislocated disk can testify. And phase-two treatment is often the only way of providing long-range relief.

Incidentally, there is at present little controversy over oral surgery, either on the joints or the jaws. It is widely recognized to be a medical procedure, to solve functional and structural problems, and is thus covered by medical insurance. Some companies used to promote the view that such surgery was purely cosmetic, because it made patients look better. The courts took a dim view of this argument, and now most medical carriers honor TMJ surgery claims without much question.

This background shows why insurance for TMJ treatment remains an uncertain and controversial area for patients, for dentists, and even for insurers. If you hope to have treatment paid for by insurance, you must be prepared to tread very carefully through what has become a procedural minefield.

• Policies and Their Pitfalls

The following information and advice apply only to TMJ disorders that are *not* the result of accidents or injuries caused by others. A very different kind of insurance, which I'll discuss later, covers accidents and injuries.

The first step in seeking insurance reimbursement, whether under a medical or dental policy, should come *before* treatment begins. You should check the policy itself and its accompanying manual carefully, especially for disorders and treatments that are specifically *excluded* from coverage—as TMJ disorders sometimes are. You may also find it helpful to seek advice from your insurance agent or from the benefits manager of your employer. Or you can seek guidance from the insurance company itself. If TMJ disorders are indeed identified for exclusion, you will probably have difficulty making a successful claim.

If you have a dental plan and hope to be reimbursed for phase-two treatment, check the policy for restrictions on orthodontics and restorative dentistry. For example, some policies exclude orthodontics performed after a certain age: they rule out treatment for adults, but TMJ disorders usually turn up in adulthood. Such policies effectively deny coverage for phase-two orthodontics.

Some policies also have a troublesome clause regarding restorative dentistry. Coverage is denied for any *replacement* of a restorative appliance—a bridge, say, or a denture—within five years of its insertion. The insurance companies maintain that if an appliance proves defective within that period, it should be the responsibility of the dentist to correct or replace it. The trouble is that phase-two treatment of TMJ problems often requires either the substantial alteration or replacement of existing appliances—something the dentist who made them could not have anticipated. Again, it is the patient who gets left out on a limb.

Finally, both dental and medical policies, almost without exception, exclude coverage for treatment of "pre-existing conditions." This is true of all insurance: you can't get life insurance once you are stricken with a fatal illness. But sometimes the exclusion is construed to deny coverage for most TMJ disorders on the grounds that they are caused by malocclusion, or by habitual grinding or clenching, that "pre-existed" before the time the policy took effect.

To be just, insurance carriers have reason to be cautious in accepting claims. Legally, once an insurer takes responsibility for one claim arising from an insured person's illness or injury, that insurer is likely to be liable for any and all other claims arising from the same condition. This can indeed become a blank check for the insured.

Most policies require, or allow the insured to select, a certain minimum amount to be deducted from claim payments. There's nothing wrong with this. It saves money for the insurer and cuts down on the premiums paid by the insured. More serious, however, are specified limits of payment for particular procedures. These may be set relatively low, and health providers aren't obliged to accept them as payment in full without advance consent.

More desirable, from the patient's point of view, are policies that agree to pay the "reasonable and customary" fees of practitioners in the region. But these represent an average and, again, no practitioner is obliged to accept them as full payment. I cannot emphasize too strongly the need to discuss costs fully, frankly, and in advance of treatment.

Dental policies often have special limits. They may set a maximum payment for any given year. Or they may set a limit on the maximum to be paid for a certain kind of procedure, such as orthodontics, over the lifetime of the insured. Both these limits may make it difficult for the patient to cover the total costs of orthodontics or other phase-two treatment.

You can sometimes cover deductibles and other payment limitations in your own policy if your spouse has a policy that also covers you. You can then apply for what is called *co-insurance*. You make a primary claim under your own policy, and on the claim form identify your spouse's policy. You then make a secondary claim under that policy. The payment may be enough to cover the deductible or other shortfall.

Insurance policies vary widely, and to a certain extent you get what you pay for. If you are selecting health insurance for yourself, it pays to shop around and to pay attention to the fine print. Most people, though, don't have the luxury of choosing for themselves—they are covered by a group policy, which considerably reduces their premiums. Usually group plans are provided by employers, but they are sometimes set up by unions or other membership organizations.

Group policies vary, too. Coverage available to upper-level executives may be considerably more liberal than what is available to entry-level employees. If you are covered by a group policy and have any choice about the extent of your coverage or the level of your own contribution, beware of what may prove to be false economies in a "bare-bones" policy.

• Submitting the Initial Claim

Despite all the cautionary information above, I nonetheless recommend that you submit any and all claims for TMJ treatment to your *medical* insurer unless the policy excludes such coverage explicity. As I've said, policies and their interpretation vary considerably.

Some practitioners have a supply of standard claim forms for carriers such as Blue Cross and Blue Shield. Usually, though, you must get a form from your agent or from your employer. You fill out part of it, then take it to the dentist or other practitioner, who will also fill out a part. Either you, your dentist, or your employer will then submit the claim to the insurer.

Many dentists have a universal, generic insurance form of their own, familiarly known as a "superbill." It lists all customary procedures, and those that have been performed are simply checked off and dated. This form is used instead of filling out the practitioner's part of the claim form. You attach it to the claim form when submitting it.

But a superbill, or any other form filled out by a dentist, can have its drawbacks when submitted to a medical insurer. You should make sure that your dentist is familiar with the particular requirements of a medical claim for TMJ procedures (any TMJ practitioner is likely to have been through the mill on this, but it's best to be certain).

For example, precise and rather special medical nomenclature must often be used. For instance, the condition that dentists know as myofascial pain dysfunction (MPD) is sometimes better described as "myositis" or "myalgia." There exist standard, numbered lists of medical nomenclature that cover both diagnosis and treatment. To avoid misunderstanding and argument over a claim, the dentist should use terms from these lists, including their numbers, in filling out the claim form. Information about a book containing these lists is included in the Appendix.

Sometimes a patient will ask me whether I will "accept assignment." This means that, instead of the patient paying for my services and then seeking reimbursement from the insurance company, I will submit the insurance claim on the patient's behalf and will then accept whatever the insurer provides as payment in full. Like most dentists, I must say no to such a request; I can't afford to do otherwise. It is, after all, the patient or the patient's group that has the contract with the insurance company.

• The Next Round

The insurance company may pay the claim as first submitted. But if the amount of the claim is large and if the treatment includes phase-two procedures, the company may seek to deny or reduce it, or at least to get further corroboration.

The first step is usually a letter from the company to the dentist or other practitioner, asking questions about some or all aspects of the diagnosis and treatment. A full *narrative report* may be required, including some or all of the following elements:

- Complete medical and dental history of the patient
- History of the disorder
- Diagnosis of the disorder, including records of all examinations and diagnostic tests, and evidence that the disorder is medical and not dental

• Detailed description of all forms of treatment employed, with evidence that the treatment is medical rather than dental in nature
• Account of treatment results and prognosis
• If treatment is not yet complete, a treatment plan for the future
• List of treatment costs already incurred and a projection of future costs

Needless to say, all health providers loathe this kind of paperwork and grumble over the burden insurance companies put on them. Nonetheless, the insurers do have good reason to insist on proof that a claim is legitimate before accepting it. Thus, your dentist should respond to such a request in a timely fashion—usually within a month. And the narrative report must be complete and accurate. If the claim is ever submitted for arbitration or becomes the subject of a lawsuit (which sometimes happens, alas), the report will become legal evidence.

The insurance company still may not be satisfied and may insist on its right to have you examined by one or more of its own consultants. Such consultants are likely to probe for reasons such as "pre-existing conditions" to justify denying the claim. If your claim is denied, you can still appeal your case. You must first do so to the claims supervisor of the insurance company. Then, in many states, you have the right to request arbitration. Otherwise, especially if the claim is substantial, you may feel you have no alternative but to seek legal counsel and sue.

• Liability and No-Fault Insurance

TMJ disorders that result from accidents, or from injuries caused by others are covered by a wholly different kind of insurance—*liability* insurance. Most liability claims arise out of motor-vehicle accidents. If you suffer a TMJ disorder as the result, say, of a whiplash injury in a collision, you will not submit a claim to your medical insurer. Instead, you will make a claim against the owner of the other vehicle, who in virtually every state must carry liability insurance to cover such claims. In recent years, many states have replaced ordinary liability insurance with *no-fault* insurance, which doesn't require the determination of responsibility for an accident and saves a lot of lawsuits.

Liability and no-fault insurance cover injuries and the disorders that result from them. Hence there is not the distinction between medical and dental conditions that muddies the water of health insurance. However, liability and no-fault insurance have their own pitfalls, further complicated by widely varying state laws.

For example, although most states with a no-fault system mandate payment of "reasonable and customary" fees, not all do. Some (such as New York) have a schedule of fixed fees for all procedures; others have fixed ceilings for total costs. In fact, if you face any substantial medical costs as a result of an accident, you will probably need the services of a lawyer to protect your interests.

TMJ disorders resulting from accidents pose at least two special insurance problems of their own. First, such disorders may not show up immediately after the accident. They may be temporarily masked by other injuries, or they may take several months to start producing painful symptoms. The insurer may then question the connection between the accident and the disorder.

The second problem is that of "pre-existing conditions." (A similar problem arises under medical insurance.) The insurer may maintain that the disorder didn't result from the accident but from a "pre-existing" physical condition, such as malocclusion or habitual clenching and grinding.

Liability insurers, like health insurers, are likely to require extensive narrative reports like those already described. The reports will include one important additional feature: The practitioner must establish a clear cause-and-effect connection between the accident and the disorders being treated.

Furthermore, the insurers may require you to be examined by their own experts. These experts are going to be skeptical of claims, to say the least. However, remember that the insurance companies have good reason to be cautious. Once they honor one claim arising out of an accident, they are liable for all further claims arising from the same event.

As a result of these various barriers and pitfalls, many people who have been injured end up suffering doubly. They suffer pain and disability from the injuries themselves, and they also suffer the psychological pain of a long and difficult struggle to collect damages. It is often necessary for patients to retain a lawyer to obtain reimbursement for their medical costs.

• Workers' Compensation

Finally, I should mention at least briefly one special form of liability insurance, which covers injuries suffered on the job. *Workers' compensation* insurance exists in virtually every state and covers a large majority of workers. It works somewhat like no-fault insurance, but it is financed by compulsory contributions from employers and employees and is administered by the state.

Instead of having to bring a lawsuit and prove negligence, an injured employee submits a claim to the state for workers' compensation. Most states have schedules of fixed payments for various kinds of injuries, but these schedules (and other limits and conditions for claims) vary widely from one state to another.

Patients making claims for TMJ problems resulting from on-the-job injuries (a fall, say, or an accident in an employer-owned vehicle) are likely to face the same difficulties as liability and no-fault claimants. Their claims may be questioned on the grounds that the condition wasn't directly caused by the injury or arose from a preexisting condition. Usually the state provides mediation and arbitration in such disputes.

You may find this whole subject of insurance rather depressing. I certainly do. It would be highly desirable if there were simple, noncontroversial ways to provide medical and liability coverage for all potential patients. The existing systems are full of confusion, conflict, and uncertainty. In my view, they cause patients unjust and unnecessary hardship, which can interfere with their recovery.

ELEVEN

A SUMMARY OF SELF-HELP

Treating TMJ disorders is mainly a job for professionals: dentists, physical therapists, psychologists, surgeons, and so forth. Nonetheless, there are several things that you can do for yourself if you have a TMJ disorder, think you may have one, or want to avoid getting one. I have discussed almost all of them in the foregoing chapters, but for your convenience I'm going to sum them up briefly here. I will address three basic questions:

- How can I tell if I have a TMJ disorder?
- What can I do to relieve symptoms and assist recovery?
- How can I reduce my chances of getting a TMJ disorder in the first place?

• How Can I Tell If I Have a TMJ Disorder?

Do-it-yourself diagnosis is unwise and sometimes dangerous. This is especially true of TMJ disorders—the "painful pretenders." Even so, certain characteristic symptoms make it wise for you to consult a TMJ practitioner:

- *Headaches*, often severe and recurrent. They tend to occur more commonly on one side than on both and in areas around the eyes, cheeks, and temples but can also occur at the top or base of the skull.
- *Toothaches* that cannot be traced to decay, nerve death, or inflammation.
- *Burning, tingling sensations*, especially in the tongue but sometimes in the mouth or throat.
- *Earaches* or "stuffed" sensations in the ears, sometimes accompanied by dizziness or by ringing or rushing noises.
- *Neckaches or shoulderaches*, sometimes accompanied by numbness in the arms or hands.
- *Tenderness and swelling*, particularly in the sides of the face.
- *Clicking or popping noises* when opening the jaw, closing it, or both.
- *Inability to open the mouth freely*, either because of pain or because some impediment seems to "lock" the jaw at a certain point. If the problem occurs on one side only, the jaw may not open straight but slides off to one side.

To obtain even stronger evidence of a possible TMJ disorder, you can perform these simple self-tests:

- Place the first two fingertips of each hand directly in front of each ear. The TMJs are directly underneath, and you should be able to feel their movement as you open and close your mouth. If even the light pressure of your fingertips causes pain on one or both sides, joint inflammation is a possibility.
- Holding your hands near the sides of your face, tip them backward so the fingertips are pointing toward you.

Place all four fingertips against the lower jaw on each side, with the forefinger near the angle of the jaw. As you open and close, you can feel the thick masseter muscles that extend diagonally from the angle to the cheekbone. Pain suggests the presence of myofascial pain dysfunction (MPD) resulting from muscle fatigue.

- Press your fingers lightly against your temples above and in front of your ears. Open and close your mouth. If you feel pain, one or both of the fan-shaped temporalis muscles may be fatigued and sore.

The following resistance tests will help you spot possible fatigue and soreness of the less accessible pterygoid muscles inside the jaws:

- With the mouth partly open, press three fingers against the lower front teeth—firmly but not hard. Then close the jaw against this resistance.
- With the jaw closed, press a fist against your chin and open against the resistance.
- Press an open palm against each side of the lower jaw in turn and move the jaw sideways against the resistance.

If any of these tests cause noticeable pain, one or more of the muscles may be fatigued and inflamed.

• What Can I Do to Relieve Symptoms and Assist Recovery?

Many of the medications and other procedures used to treat TMJ disorders must be administered by professionals. But you can obtain certain effective pain relievers over the counter, and you can undertake some forms of physical therapy and psychological training on your own. And you can certainly change certain physical habits, such as posture—changes that can make you feel better and assist in your eventual recovery.

Medications should be used sparingly and not over a long period. Otherwise they tend to hide the disorder rather than cure it. But I see no harm in them when used to relieve acute pain, and some of them need no prescription.

- *Aspirin* is a very effective analgesic (painkiller), with coated forms available for those with sensitive stomachs. Aspirin also helps reduce inflammation in muscle and joint tissues.
- Most anti-inflammatory medications require a prescription, but *ibuprofen* is available over the counter in very mild form under the trade name Advil. Taken as instructed, it may relieve pain, but it won't be strong enough to control inflammation. And it isn't safe for you to take larger doses without professional supervision.
- Salves and sprays containing *local anesthetics* can give temporary relief to sore muscles like the masseter and temporalis. Be careful to keep them away from your eyes.

One way to control the pain of inflammation is not to take something but to *avoid* something. That something is caffeine. It stimulates the central nervous system, increases muscle tension, and increases sensitivity to pain. The strongest source is coffee, but tea, chocolate, and cola drinks also contain it.

I often encourage patients to make at least temporary use of what I call "walking-cane" therapies. These give inflamed TMJs or sore chewing muscles a rest, just as a cane rests a twisted ankle or strained knee.

- *Limit jaw movement.* Open your jaws only as far as you feel no pain, and avoid wide opening. If you feel a yawn coming on, restrict it by pressing a fist under your chin.

• *Soft diet.* You don't have to switch entirely to liquids and baby food. But avoid foods like raw vegetables, nuts, hard rolls, and chewy meat such as steak. Also chewing gum.

For main dishes use pasta and noodles as well as casseroles and hashes made with chopped or minced meat, fish, or eggs. Substitute cooked vegetables and fruits for raw. For dessert stick to puddings, custards, and ice cream, which give little or no work to the joints or their surrounding muscles.

See the Appendix for information on the *Non-Chew Cookbook*, designed to keep patients on soft diets from dying of dietary boredom.

There are a few forms of physical therapy you can use on your own, both to ease pain and restore function.

Heat and cold are old but effective remedies for relieving pain and reducing inflammation. Some patients respond better to one than the other, and some are helped most by the use of the two in succession.

• Methods of heat application include the *moist compress*, a towel or other absorbent fabric soaked in hot water. A hot-water bottle applied over the compress will keep it warm longer. Also available are professional devices such as the Hydrocolator, available at hospital-supply stores and some drugstores. It contains a fluid-filled plastic pouch which is inserted into a fabric wrapper held in place with Velcro fasteners.

• The simplest way to apply cold is in the form of *ice*. I recommend sealing it in a plastic bag, which is then wrapped in a dry cloth. You can also use a ready-made *cold pack*, which remains flexible even when chilled below the freezing temperature of water. A *snap-pack* doesn't even have to be chilled. Striking it on a hard surface sets off a chemical reaction that makes it lose heat quickly.

Caution: Don't apply ice for more than about twenty minutes in any hour or you can damage your skin.

Physical therapists often instruct TMJ patients in special exercises designed to give greater flexibility to the muscles of the head and neck. A short series of these is outlined in Chapter 6 on page 103.

Just as important are efforts to correct bad posture and other physical habits that contribute to TMJ disorders and interfere with recovery. These include:

• The *forward-positioned head,* with the head thrust forward, and the chin tilted up. Sometimes called "bird-watcher's posture," this is the most harmful of postural faults. The weight of your head puts undesirable pressure on the neck and back muscles and also strains the TMJs themselves.

• *Poor standing posture.* There is more to good posture than simply "standing up straight." An exaggerated military posture, chest thrust forward and chin up, is almost as harmful as a forward slump. Your chest and shoulders should be relaxed and your head balanced at the top of your neck, your chin tucked in.

You can assure good standing posture by using the natural weight distribution of your body. Instead of standing with your weight concentrated over your heels, rock forward slightly so your weight is mainly on the balls of your feet. As the weight of your lower body shifts forward, your head and shoulders will naturally settle back to serve as a balancing counterweight.

• *Poor sitting posture.* Many chairs don't support the middle and lower back, but instead encourage slumping. You can insert a small cushion between your back and the chair to provide the missing support. It also helps not to sit cross-legged or to sit for a long time in one position without a break.

When you drive, make sure the seat isn't too far back, or too low in relationship to the dashboard, so that you have to crane forward to see the road. If the seat won't adjust sufficiently, extra cushions behind or under you can sometimes make up the difference.

• *Poor lying posture.* The worst fault is lying on your stomach with your head twisted to one side. Almost as bad is lying on your back with your head propped up at a sharp angle for reading or watching television. The healthiest and most restful lying position is on the side, with a pillow thick enough to support the head and neck horizontally and the arms and legs loosely flexed.

• *Other positions and habits to avoid:*

—Cradling the telephone between shoulder and chin

—Propping the chin on one or both hands for extended periods

—Reaching high overhead for burdens; also painting, hammering, or doing other work on high walls or ceilings

—Carrying a heavy shoulder bag with the strap on the same shoulder for an extended period

—Wearing high-heeled boots or shoes

Often the most effective form of posture re-education is simply increased awareness. Once you're aware of the problem, it is usually not difficult to correct it. At first, you may only correct the unhealthy habit when you're thinking about it, but gradually this conscious correction will become translated into a new, healthy habit.

One bad physical habit that's extremely hard to get rid of is the most harmful of all: clenching or grinding the teeth, widely believed to be a major cause of TMJ disorders. Unless it is overcome, full recovery is unlikely.

You can fight the habit by trying to keep your mouth in what we call the "healthy resting position." Open your jaw slightly, so the upper and lower teeth are separated. Rest your tongue lightly against the roof of your mouth without pressing against the front teeth. Keep your lips shut so that you breathe through your nose.

With practice, this position may itself become a habit, reducing the urge to clench or grind. But it may desert you in stressful life situations by day, and at night, too, if you grind in your sleep. To overcome clenching and grinding, it is often necessary to retrain your body's whole response to stress.

There are many forms of professional stress therapy, ranging from psychotherapy to biofeedback. But there are a few simple physical and mental exercises that you can try on your own:

- A *breathing exercise.* This serves as an "instant tranquilizer" and can be practiced anywhere, any time.
  - —Inhale slowly and deeply, counting up to five at one-second intervals. Between each count, think of a single word (such as *calm* or *peace*) to help free your mind of distracting or stressful thoughts.
  - —Hold your breath for one second, then exhale slowly, counting backward from five to one, and silently repeat your chosen word. At the same time, let your chest and stomach muscles relax, and drop your shoulders.
  - —Repeat this cycle three times.
- *Progressive relaxation* exercises. You tense and then relax groups of related muscles in progression, over the whole body. There is no set order, but you might start with the hands (making a fist), proceed to the feet (curling the toes), and end at the head (wrinkling the forehead). Tensing the muscles before relaxing them seems to produce a greater degree of relaxation than just trying to relax them.

Directions for a complete set of progressive relaxation exercises appear in Chapter 7, on pages 118-121.

• *Guided imagery*. This technique induces relaxation by calling up to "the mind's eye" a series of soothing sensory images. You develop a mental image of a pleasant, tranquil experience to which you consciously guide your attention. At first this method is used just for training, to reduce emotional tension. But, like breathing exercise or progressive relaxation, it eventually becomes habitual and can be used to provide relief in stressful life situations.

A typical scenario for guided imagery appears in Chapter 7 on page 112.

• How Can I Reduce My Chances of Getting a TMJ Disorder in the First Place?

The exact causes of TMJ disorders are still not completely understood, so it is impossible to say that doing certain things, or not doing others, will surely keep you from getting such a disorder. Nonetheless, evidence points to two conditions that at least predispose people to TMJ problems. One is malocclusion; the other is clenching and grinding the teeth.

I have already described techniques to overcome clenching and grinding. I cannot overemphasize the importance of ridding yourself of these destructive habits. Not only are they strongly implicated in TMJ disorders such as disk displacement, but they cause severe and lasting damage to your teeth.

The best defense against malocclusion is to take care of your teeth. A common cause of malocclusion is teeth lost, as a result of poor care of the teeth and gums. Yet modern techniques make it likely—not just possible—that you can retain your natural teeth in good working order for your whole life.

Follow your dentist's advice. Brush regularly, and use dental floss and gum stimulators. Make sure your children receive fluoride treatments or use a fluoride toothpaste. Have your teeth checked and professionally cleaned twice a year, and don't let tooth decay or gum inflammation go untreated.

A question may have occurred to you: if restorative dentistry and orthodontics are so useful in stabilizing TMJ treatment, should they be used to *prevent* TMJ disorders? Based on present knowledge, the answer is: not for that reason *alone*. True, these techniques can and do remedy malocclusion, and malocclusion is implicated in TMJ disorders. But many people with even severe malocclusion never come down with TMJ disorders. Also, some people with sound teeth and good bites nonetheless develop these problems.

There are plenty of good reasons to undertake restorative dentistry or orthodontics. Appearance is one; another is a comfortable and efficient bite. But the evidence doesn't justify either procedure as a way to head off TMJ disorders.

Finally, there is one other, indisputable cause of TMJ disorders, or at least a triggering circumstance: physical injury to the jaws. This usually results from accidents, especially auto accidents. So one of the things you can do to avoid TMJ disorders—and many other problems as well—is follow safety procedures at home and drive safely and defensively on the road.

APPENDIX OF RESOURCES

Professional organizations to which TMJ practitioners are likely to belong:

American Equilibration Society
8726 North Ferris Avenue
Morton Grove, IL 60053
Telephone: (312) 965-2888

American Academy of Craniomandibular Disorders
Martha Boam, Executive Secretary
10 Joplin Court
Lafayette, CA 94549
(To receive membership list, enclose a stamped, self-addressed envelope.)

American Academy of Head, Facial, and Neck Pain and TMJ Orthopedics
Medical Towers Building
Suite 803
255 South 17th Street
Philadelphia, PA 19103
Telephone: (215) 545-2100

Cookbook and nutritional guide for patients on soft diets:

The Non-Chew Cookbook
J. Randy Wilson, ed.
Wilson Publishing
Box 2190
Glenwood Springs, CO 81602
Telephone: (303) 945-5600

Professional associations of psychologists engaged in behavioral therapy and biofeedback:

Association for Advancement of Behavioral Therapy
15 West 36th Street
New York, NY 10018
Telephone: (212) 279-7970

Biofeedback Society of America
10200 West 44th Avenue

Suite 304
Wheat Ridge, CO 80033
Telephone: (303) 422-8436

Professional associations of orthodontists:

American Association of Orthodontists
460 North Lindbergh
St. Louis, MO 63141

Professional associations of oral surgeons and practitioners of arthroscopic surgery:

American Association of Oral and Maxillofacial Surgeons
9700 Bryn Mawr Avenue
Rosemont, IL 60018
Telephone: (800) 822-6637

International Study Group for TMJ Arthroscopy
Orthopedic Institute, HIJD-OI
Department of Orthopedic Surgery
301 East 17th Street
Suite 1410
New York, NY 10003

Sources of standard terminology for insurance reports:

Current Procedural Terminology
American Medical Association
535 North Dearborn Street
Chicago, IL 60610

ICD-9
Box 971
Ann Arbor, MI 48106

INDEX
